AF539829

Pig Production and Management

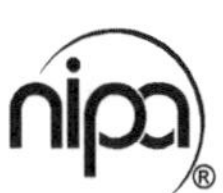

NIPA® GENX ELECTRONIC RESOURCES & SOLUTIONS P. LTD.
New Delhi-110 034

About the Author

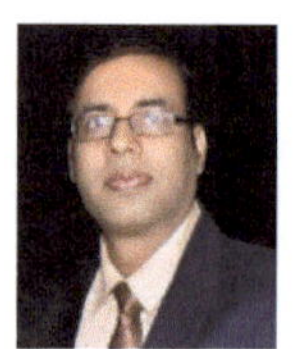

Dr. Vijay Kumar, B.V.Sc. & A.H. (CCSHAU, Hisar), M.V.Sc. and Ph.D. (Animal Genetics & Breeding), National Dairy Research Institute, Karnal, Assistant Professor in Department of Animal Genetics and Breeding at U.P. Pt. Deen Dayal Upadhyaya Pashu Chikitsa Vigyan Vishwavidyalaya Evam Go Anusandhan Sansthan, Mathura, Uttar Pradesh, India, has been closely associated with teaching Animal Genetics and Breeding since 2011. He has published four books and two book chapters on his subject. He has also published more than 60 research and review papers in reputed national and international scientific journals. He is the recipient of Director's Medal and academic excellence Award in Ph.D. He is time to time appearing on Doordarshan DD Kisan National channel for livestock related discussion.

Pig Production and Management

Vijay Kumar
Assistant Professor
Department of Animal Genetics & Breeding
College of Veterinary Science & A.H.
U.P. Pt. Deen Dayal Upadhyaya Pashu Chikitsa Vigyan Vishwavidyalaya
Evam Go Anusandhan Sansthan
Mathura, Uttar Pradesh

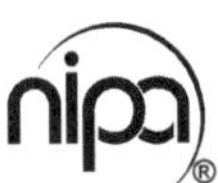

NIPA® GENX ELECTRONIC RESOURCES & SOLUTIONS P. LTD.
New Delhi-110 034

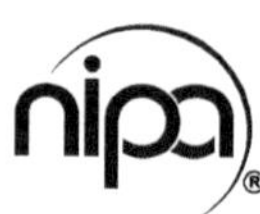

NIPA® GENX ELECTRONIC RESOURCES & SOLUTIONS P. LTD.

101,103, Vikas Surya Plaza, CU Block
L.S.C.Market, Pitam Pura, New Delhi-110 034
Ph : +91 11 27341616, 27341717, 27341718
E-mail:newindiapublishingagency@gmail.com
www: www.nipabooks.com

For customer assistance, please contact
Phone: + 91-11-27 34 17 17
Fax: + 91-11-27 34 16 16
E-Mail: feedbacks@nipabooks.com

ISBN: 978-93-95763-77-6

Composed and Designed by NIPA.

Preface

In the vast landscape of animal agriculture, one creature has proven to be an exceptional source of sustenance and livelihood: the pig. Throughout history, pigs have held a significant place in our societies, providing meat, economic stability, and a way of life for many individuals. This book, "Pig Production and Management," delves into the intricacies of pig farming, exploring its rich history, the benefits it offers, and the essential aspects of successfully managing a pig farm.

Part I of this book delves into the fascinating world of pig farming in India, tracing its origins and development over the years. Author explores the economic significance of pig farming, uncovering its evolution from traditional practices to modern techniques. Understanding the historical context of pig farming in India provides a foundation for comprehending the challenges and opportunities that exist in the present-day industry.

Part II focuses on the undeniable benefits of pig farming. Author discusses the nutritional value of pork, its contribution to food security, and its economic potential. Additionally, author explores the various by-products that can be derived from pigs, highlighting the sustainable and holistic nature of pig farming. Through this exploration, author aims to shed light on the immense value that pig farming brings to individuals, communities, and the larger livestock sector.

Part III delves into the diverse breeds of pigs found in India and in foreign countries. Author examines their characteristics, strengths, and suitability for different farming systems. By understanding the specific traits of each breed, farmers can make informed decisions regarding breeding stock and optimize their production outcomes. This section serves as a comprehensive guide to help readers navigate the intricacies of breed selection in pig farming.

Part IV focuses on the reproductive system of pigs, exploring topics such as artificial insemination and reproduction management. Author delves into the physiology of pig reproduction, providing valuable insights into breeding cycles, gestation, and parturition. Understanding these processes is crucial for successful breeding programs and efficient reproduction management on pig farms.

Part V addresses the vital aspect of breeding management. Author delves into the various mating systems employed in pig farming, considering factors such as genetic diversity, production goals, and resource optimization. Moreover, author emphasizes the importance of selecting suitable breeding stock, highlighting the key traits and characteristics to look for when building a productive and healthy pig population.

Part VI delves into the housing systems for pigs, offering insights into the design and management of pig housing facilities. Author explores the different types of housing, considering factors such as space requirements, ventilation, and waste management. By implementing appropriate housing systems, farmers can ensure the well-being and productivity of their pigs.

Part VII focuses on the digestive system of pigs and the essential role of nutrition in their growth and development. Author discusses the nutritional requirements of pigs at various life stages, exploring the formulation of balanced diets and the utilization of feed resources. Understanding the intricacies of pig nutrition is vital for optimizing growth rates, reproductive performance, and overall herd health.

Part VIII provides comprehensive guidance on pig farm management. Author covers essential topics such as record-keeping, biosecurity measures and herd health management. This section equips readers with the knowledge and tools necessary to run a successful and profitable pig farm, emphasizing the importance of effective planning, monitoring, and decision-making.

Lastly, in Part IX, author delves into the common diseases that affect pigs. Author discusses preventive measures, vaccination protocols, and the identification and management of various ailments. By understanding the potential health challenges faced by pig farmers, they can implement appropriate disease prevention and control strategies, safeguarding the well-being of their animals and ensuring the long-term sustainability of their operations.

Author is highly thankful to Prof. A K Srivastava, Vice Chancellor, DUVASU, Mathura for his continuous motivation. Author is also thankful to the students and teachers who have read my earlier four books on Animal Genetics & Breeding and encouraged me to write a book on pig production and management. Author is also highly thankful to family members – mother, wife, son and elder brothers & sister.

In compiling this comprehensive guide on pig production and management, author aims to provide a valuable resource for aspiring and seasoned pig farmers alike. It is my hope that the knowledge contained within these pages will empower readers

Author

Contents

1

Brief History of Pig Farming in India

Pig farming is considered as a beneficial sector in India that provides avenues of fast economic growth for new entrepreneurs and socioeconomically weaker sections, due to high fecundity rate, better-feed conversion efficiency, early maturity, small generation interval, and minimum investment on housing and equipment. Pig farming has evolved into a semi-commercial enterprise using intensive farming practises, in addition to being reared through free range management. Pig farming provides money to rural impoverished people from the lowest socioeconomic strata. As a result, effective programmes to popularise technological pig rearing of meat producing animals with enough financial supplies are required to modernise the Indian pig business and advance the productivity of small sized rural pig farms. Given the importance of pig farming in terms of its interaction with the rural poor and the potential for pig rearing in our country, the Government of India has launched initiatives to support scientific pig farming through its five-year plans. Regional pig breeding facilities were constructed to make solid foundation stock available. The majority of pigs in India are indigenous breeds, while the population of cross-bred and exotic pigs has expanded. Hampshire, Large White York Shire, Duroc, Landrace, and Tamworth are among the exotic breeds, while Ghungroo, Niang Megha, Ankamali, Agonda Goan, and Tany-Vo are among the prominent indigenous pig breeds. Native breeds are small, slow growing, have fewer litters, and produce low-quality meat. The average meat yield of native breeds in India is roughly 35 kg/animal, which is lower than the global average of around 78 kg/animal. To improve piggery production and overcome the poor performance of local pig germplasm, India imported exotic pigs such as Duroc, Berkshires, Hampshire, Landrace, Large White Yorkshire, Saddleback, and Tamworth. Various crossbred pigs were also developed by research institutes by crossing local pigs with exotic breeds to generate animals with much improved output and superior qualities.

Pig population

The global pig population has been estimated to reach 784.20 million. According to the data from the 20th Livestock Census, India has a total of 9.06

million pigs. Between the 10th (1966) and 11th (1972) Livestock Censuses, the pig population increased dramatically as a result of a variety of breeding programmes that raised awareness of the benefits of piggery farming. Later, beginning in 2003, a downward trend in the pig population was noted. According to the 20th Livestock Census, the pig population in India's major pig producing states (Assam, Jharkhand, Meghalaya, West Bengal, Chhattisgarh, Uttar Pradesh, Nagaland, Bihar, Karnataka, and Mizoram) improved from the previous livestock census.

Indigenous pigs

In India, indigenous pigs account for around 79.03% of the pig population. The National Bureau of Animal Genetic Resources has documented ten indigenous pigs in India: Agonda Goan, Doom, Ghoongroo, Gurrah, Mali, Niang Megha, Nicobari, Purnea, Tenyi-Vo, and Zovawk. These pig breeds are raised by farmers spread over the country. They are smaller and better adaptable to poor weather conditions. Most importantly, they have improved disease resistance, which is critical in livestock farming. Although these breeds have enhanced disease resistance, their production performance is notably low when compared to foreign breeds. As a result, exotic breeds have been imported to improve output performance. The eastern and north eastern states have the highest pig population (72.21%), followed by northern southern (10.68%), central (7.64%), northern (6.79%), and western India (2.69%). Assam has the most population (2.10 million), followed by Jharkhand (1.28 million), Meghalaya (0.70 million), and West Bengal (0.54 million). Indigenous pigs (79.03%) form the foundation of the country's pork industry, followed by crossbred and exotic germplasm (20.95%). Although the pig population has decreased (12.03%) since the last census, the population in the major pig producing states has increased.

Genetic Improvement Programmes

Year	Milestone
Pre independence	Christian missionaries bring some pigs from foreign countries
1948	Base Pig Breeding Farms (BPBF) were established in Khanapara, Guwahati introduced Large black, Berkshire and Saddle back
1970-71	AICRP on Pig was established to assess production, reproduction and efficiency of feed utilization. Tirupati & Jabbalpur : Large White Yorkshire Khanapara & Izzatnagar : Landrace
1976	National Commission on Agriculture recommend crossbreeding of local pigs with AICRP centers
1976	Hampshire was imported 30-Sow unit, Khanapara, BPBF-Khanapara and Barapani (Meghalaya)

1978	Large white Yorkshire was introduced in AICRP centers
1988	Imported LWH, Landrace and Saddle back
2002	Imported Hampshire and gave it to Assam, Meghalaya and Arunachal Pradesh.

Major central sponsored breeding programmes

- All India Coordinated Research Project on Pigs (started in 1970-71)
- Mega seed project (started in 2008-09)
- National Livestock Mission

All India Coordinated Research Project (AICRP) on Pig: began during the Fourth Five Year Plan (1970-1971) with the primary purpose of reviewing purebred performance. The significant necessity for upgrading native pigs was recognised towards the end of the Fifth Five Year Plan due to their socioeconomic relevance. As a result, in order to provide a constructive approach in pig production, the AICRP Pig Technical Programme was completely redesigned at the start of the Sixth Five Year Plan to conduct research on indigenous pigs and then on crossbreeding between indigenous and acceptable exotic breeds.

AICRP on Pigs center

S.No.	Name of the center
1	College of Veterinary Science, Assam Agricultural University
2	College of Veterinary & Animal Science, Kerala Veterinary and Animal Science University
3	Sri Venkateshwara Veterinary University, Tirupati
4	ICAR-Central Coastal Agricultural Research Institute, Ela, Goa
5	Indian Veterinary Research Institute, Izatnagar
6	Tamil Nadu Veterinary and Animal Sciences University, Kattupakkam
7	College of Veterinary Science &AH, CAU, Selesih, Aizawl
8	SASARD, Medziphema, Nagaland
9	ICAR-Central Island Agricultural Research Institute, Garacharama, Port Blair
10	College of Agriculture, CAU, Iroisemba, Imphal
11	ICAR Research Complex for NEH Region, Umroi Road, Umiam
12	Indian Veterinary Research Institute (IVRI), Eastern Regional Station (ERS), Kolkata

13	KVK Goalpara, Dudhnoi,
14	Krantisinh Nana Patil College of Veterinary Science, (Maharashtra Animal and Fishery Sciences University), Shirval
15	College of Veterinary Science, Guru Angad Dev Veterinary and Animal Sciences University, Ludhiana

Mega seed project on pigs

The mega-seed project on pig was established by ICAR in 2008. National Research Centre on Pig is managing the Mega-seed Project on Pig. The project has four centers as follows:

- Assam Agricultural University, Khanapara
- Birsa Agricultural University, Ranchi
- ICAR RC for NEH, Nagaland Centre, Medziphema
- State Veterinary Department, Aizawl, Mizoram

The project was launched with an aim to generate and provide superior swine germplasm to the local farmers. In XIIth five year plan an additional four centers were approved for Mega Seed Project on Pig as follows:

- State Animal Husbandry and Veterinary Department, Govt. of Arunachal Pradesh
- Kerala Veterinary and Animal Science University, Pookode, Kerala
- Animal Resource Development Department, Govt. of Tripura, Agartala, Tripura
- Chhattisgarh Kamdhenu Vishwavidyalaya, Durg, Chhattisgarh

National Livestock Mission

The National Livestock Mission (NLM), which was initiated in 2014-15, aims to strengthen livestock production systems and increase capacity for all stakeholders. The plan focuses on entrepreneurial growth and breed enhancement in poultry, sheep, goats, and pigs, as well as feed and fodder development. Pig farming is gradually capturing the attention of livestock producers in India, who have realised the value of these animals as moneymakers. Experts in animal husbandry see the increase in pig population as astonishing. Pig farming is more profitable than goat or cattle husbandry, especially when well managed. Pigs are more prolific than cows or goats. The sector is not without its difficulties, particularly in the handling of disease outbreaks.

SWOT Analysis of Piggery in India

Strength

- High income and profitability
- Pig farms can be built on small areas, and feed costs are much lower.
- The demand for pork meat has grown throughout time.
- Regulatory compliance is uncomplicated.
- The production time is shorter than that of red meat.

Weakness

- Societal taboos
- Breed upgradation is low, and concentrate feed is unavailable.
- Weak supply chain/marketing infrastructure.
- Meat processing infrastructure is more labour intensive.

Opportunities

- Increasing demand
- Export and value addition
- Medium for poverty reduction.
- Self-employment
- An industry with enormous growth potential.

Threats

- Diseases such as ASF
- Volatile cost and revenue
- Regulations
- Highly subjected to global conditions and inexpensive imports.

2

Benefits of Pig Farming

The issues that our country faces in ensuring nutritional security for its rapidly growing population necessitate an integrated strategy to domestic animal rearing. Of the various livestock species, pigs are the most likely source of meat production and the most capable feed converters after broiler chickens. It not only provides meat but also bristles and dung. Pig farming provides rural residents with job options and additional revenue to help them better their living conditions. It is critical to assist capital formation in the animal husbandry sector in order to boost farmer incomes. The following are the benefits of pig farming:

- The feed conversion efficiency of the pig is best possible. Except for broilers, pigs produce more live weight gain per kg of feed than any other class of meat-producing animals.
- The pig can transform a wide variety of feed stuffs, such as grains, forages, and broken feeds into valuable nutritious meat. Furthermore, the majority of these meals are not edible or pleasing to humans.
- They reproduce quickly and have a short generation interval. A sow can be bred at the age of 8-9 months and farrow twice a year. Each farrowing produces 6-12 piglets.
- Buildings and equipment investment is very low for pig farming.
- Pigs are noted for their meat production, which ranges from 65-80% in terms of dressing percentage, in contrast to other livestock species, whose dressing yields may not exceed 65%.
- Pig excrement is often utilised as a fertiliser in agricultural and fish ponds.
- Pigs quickly acquire fat, which is in high demand from the poultry feed, soap, paint, and other chemical industries.
- Pig farming gives quick returns because the profitable weight of fatteners can be obtained in 6-8 months.
- The farmer can profitably utilise his time and labour in this activity with a small investment in building and equipment, proper feeding, and a strong disease management programme.

- Pig - Horti - Agri - Pasture - Sylvi - Fish farming are the best options for an integrated farming system.
- Pork is a relatively inexpensive animal protein source. Pig products range from raw commodities like pork to processed delicacies like sausages and smoked hams to roasted salted ears consumed as snacks.
- Pork is particularly healthy because of its high fat and low water content, and it has a higher energy value than other meats. It contains vitamins such as thiamin, niacin, and riboflavin.
- Pig products such as pork, bacon, ham, sausages, lard, and so on are in high demand both domestically and internationally.

3

Pig Breeds

The indigenous pig has been the basis used for pig production for a long period of time. It is small in size. Improved breeds are now being used for grading up the form the basis for pig production in the rural areas. The majority of the pig population in India is of indigenous breeds though population of cross-bred and exotic pigs increased by 12.7 percent from year 2003 to 2012. The exotic breed mainly comprises Hampshire, Large White York Shire, Duroc, Landrace, and Tamworth.

Exotic Pig Breeds

The important exotic pig breeds are as follows

Large white Yorkshire

- Most extensively used exotic breed in India
- Body colour is solid white
- Erect ears, snout of medium lengths and dished face
- Excellent breed for the purpose of cross breeding
- Prolific breeds
- Mature boar 300-400 kg
- Mature sow 230-320 kg
- The large white Yorkshire is native breed of United Kingdom and is reported to produce better bacon when crossed with other suitable types.
- This breed was imported into India frm UK, New Zealand and Australia.
- Skin is pink colored and is free form wrinkles with long and moderately fine coat.
- Neck is long and full to the shoulder with deep and wide chest.
- Back is slightly arched; loin is long and broad with a well developed wide rump.
- Tail is set high.
- This breed is very popular for the bacon.

Landrace

- Body colour is white
- Long body, large drooping ears and long snout
- Prolific breeding and efficient in utilizing feed
- Carcass quality equal to Yorkshire
- Excellent breed for crossbreeding
- Mature boars weigh 270-360 kg
- Mature sow weighs 200-320 kg
- There has to be a high proportion of lean meat and a small proportion of fat and fine bone.
- The carcass of this breed is so proportioned that as much as possible could be made into bacon with as little wastage as possible.
- Sows have good mothering quality.

Middle white Yorkshire

- Grows rapidly gives good dressing percentage
- Not so prolific as large white Yorkshire
- Males 250-340 kg
- Females 180-270 kg
- The middle While Yorkshire was evolved as a result of crossing Large White Yorkshire and Small Yorkshire breeds of UK.
- It is a medium sized bacon pig and a good porker at light weights.
- It is white in colour with a short head unturned dished face wide between the ears.
- Neck is blended neatly from head and to shoulder.
- Ears are nearly erect but somewhat inclined forwards.
- Hams are broad and fleshy upto the hocks.

Berkshire

- The Berkshire is one of the oldest English breed of swine.
- This breed is valued as producer of quality meat, especially suitable for the pork market.
- This breed is used in upgrading programs.

- The pigs are black with white markings usually on the feet, head and tail.
- It has a short head with dished face.
- The snout is short.
- The body is long and ribs well sprung.
- Mature boars weigh about 280-360 kg or more.

Hampshire

- Hampshire breed was developed in USA from hogs imported form UK.
- It is a black hog with a white belt encircling the body and including the front legs.
- Head and tail are black, and the ears are erect.
- The pigs are short legged.
- Sows are very prolific breeders.
- The weight of a mature boar is 300 kg and sow 280 kg.

Tamworth

- Tamworth is the purest modern representative of the native English pig.
- The colour is reddish or chestnut, typically golden red hairs on a flesh coloured skin. The snout is very long and straight.
- The ears are fairly large and rigid and incline forward.
- It has a strong back and thin shoulders.
- The carcass produces bacon of best quality.
- Sows are prolific breeders.
- Mature boars weigh up to 300 kg.

Duroc

- Duroc has its origin in USA.
- It is red in colour, with the shades varying form golden to very dark red.
- It is a large breed with excellent feeding capacity and prolificacy.
- The sows are good mothers.
- The weight of mature boar is 410 kg and sow 250 kg.

Wessex Saddle Back

- The Wessex Saddleback pig is a breed of domestic pig originating England.
- It is also known as Wessex pig.
- Wessex Saddleback pigs are tall animals.
- They are mainly black in color with a white band about the forepart of the trunk, extending from one fore-foot over the shoulder to the other.
- White coloration of this pig breed form a white band resembling a saddle or sheet.

Poland China

- The Poland China is an American breed of domestic pig.
- Its origins lie in a small number of pigs of Chinese type bought in 1816, which were cross-bred with a variety of breeds of European origin including the Berkshire.
- It was bred as a lard pig, and is among the largest of all pig breeds.
- The Poland China usually displays the coloration of the Berkshire: solid black, with white points on the nose, tail and feet.
- It is a large pig, heavy-jowled, lop-eared and short-legged.

Chester White

- The Chester White is a breed of domestic pig which originated in Chester County, Pennsylvania.
- The Chester White is a versatile breed suited to both intensive and extensive husbandry.
- Though not as popular as the Duroc, Yorkshire, or Hampshire, the Chester White is actively used in commercial crossbreeding operations for pork.
- Their pale colour leaves Chester Whites prone to sunburn; they must be given access to shade in the summer.

Large Black

- The Large Black pig is a British breed of domestic pig. It is the only British pig that is entirely black.
- The Large Black is a long, deep-bodied pig, well known for its hardiness and suitability for extensive farming.

- Large Blacks are best suited for pasture-based farming due to their strong foraging and grazing ability, which efficiently converts poor quality feed into meat.
- It is the only pig breed in Britain to be all black, and this helps protect the pig from sunburn in sunny climates.
- Temperamentally, the Large Black is a very docile breed which is easily contained by fencing.
- This is partly because its large, drooping ears obscure its vision, although they also help to protect the face and eyes while the animal is foraging, especially when rooting in dirt.
- The breed is also known for its long periods of fertility and strong maternal instincts.
- Sows give birth to a large litter of 8–10 piglets, but some sows have been known to have litters of up to 13 piglets.

Hereford

- The Hereford, often called the Hereford Hog, is a breed of domestic pig named for its colour and pattern, which is similar to that of the Hereford breed of cattle: red with a white face.
- Originating in the United States, the Hereford is a rare variety of swine which was created from a synthesis of Duroc, Poland China, and perhaps some Chester White or Hampshire.
- It is a pig of medium size: mature sows weigh about 270 kg and boars about 360 kg.
- The only allowable coat coloration is a deep red-brown covering at least two thirds of the body, with a pale face, ears, underbelly, and socks.
- The ears hang forwards over the face.
- It is hardy and docile, prolific and suitable to either extensive or intensive management.

Indian pig breed

Some of the popular indigenous pig breeds include Ghungroo, Niang Megha, Ankamali, Agonda Goan, and Tany-Vo.

Niang Megha

- Black, star shaped white patches at forehead and sometime hock joint
- Niang Megha is native pig of Meghalaya state

- Long tapering snout, partially white at nostril,
- long bristle on midline but uniform in other places, short ears,
- Top line-Straight in male, concave in female.

Agonda Goan

- The Agonda pig, which is native of Goa, has a capacity to adapt to hot and humid climate.
- It comes from a pure local breed, has high resistance to disease, low fat content, which people prefer in meat and early sexual maturity
- Black, few animals with white patches on leg and face
- Small bodysize, medium and rough bristle,
- slightly concave top line,
- Well adapted to local coastal environment.

Tenyi Vo

- The Native Naga pig, or tenyi vo as it is called locally, is found in Nagaland, in the extreme northeastern corner of India, along the border with Myanmar
- Colour: Black
- These are potbellied animals with sagging back and pendulous belly in females
- Straight tail ending with white marking reaching the hock joint.

Nicobari

- Nicobari pigs are semi-feral in nature and no systematic management is followed by the tribes.
- The pigs are reared under free-range system.
- Pigs are not reared for commercial purposes.
- Colour: Black, grey, brown, blakish brown and fawn skin colour.
- Marked bristle crest on the back extending from mid head/shoulder to base of the tail
- No curling is the characteristic feature of the tail.
- They are fast runner.

Doom

- These are black in colour.
- Doom is native pig of Assam state
- This pig breed is well known for meat quality and bristle.
- Top line is straight with long bristles extneding up to thoraco-lumber area.

Zovawk

- Black with white spot on forehead, white patches on belly and white boots.
- Zovawk is native pig of Mizoram state
- Long bristles on mid-line are characteristics of the Zovawk pig.
- Back: Concave top line is also characteristics of the Zovawk pig.
- Pot belly

Ghurrah

- These are black colored medium-sized pigs with a flat belly, angular body, and long straight snout.
- Ghurrah is native pig of Uttar Pradesh state
- Legs below the hock joint are white.
- Thick line of hairs is present from neck to shoulders.
- Head is elongated with triangular face and short leaf-shaped vertically erected ears.

Purnea

- Purnea is a black colored medium sized pig found in Purnea and Katihar districts of Bihar and adjoining areas of Sahibganj district of Jharkhand.
- These pigs have compact body and pot belly.
- However, in few animals, white spots at the lower limbs are also seen.
- Thick line of bristle is present on topline from neck to shoulders giving the animal a wild look.
- Animals are characterized with round face; short conical and erect ears; and small, thick and slightly concave snout.
- Skin is thick with neck folds in mature animals.
- Adult body weight varies from 41 to 50kg.
- Litter size at birth varies from 4 to 6.
- These pigs are ferocious in nature.

Ghungroo

- Ghungroo an indigenous pig first reported from North Bengal is popular among the local people because of high prolificacy and ability to sustain in low input system.
- This breed produces high quality pork utilizing agricultural byproducts and kitchen wastes.
- Ghungroo are mostly black coloured with typical 'Bull dog' face appearance, with a litter size of 6-12 piglets, individually weigh about 1.0 kg at birth and 7.0 – 10.0 kg at weaning.
- Both sexes are very much docile and easy to handle.
- In the breeding tract they are maintained under scavenging system and mainly act as insurance to the rainfed agriculture.
- Some of the selected sows have delivered litter size of 17 piglets at birth as compared to the other indigenous strains of pigs maintained at the Institute farm.

Banda Pig

- Banda pig is native of Jharkhand, mainly reared for pork and manure.
- Animals are black coloured, having short and erect ear.
- These animals are having medium to short bristle on neck with a long and concave snout.
- Average adult body weight is 28.0 kg in male and 27.0 kg in females.
- Litter size ranges from 4 to 7.

Manipuri Black

- Manipuri Black is native pig of Manipur state, mainly reared for meat.
- Adult body weight averages about 96.0 kg in males and 93.0 kg in females.
- Litter size ranges from 6 to 11 at birth.
- Meat is preferred for its taste by local people.

Wak Chambil

- Wak Chambil is a small sized pig with round and pendulous belly.
- It is mainly distributed in Garo Hills of Meghalaya.
- Pork is known for its unique flavour and taste and cherished during religious and ceremonial occasions by local people.
- Average adult body weight is 32.0 kg in males.
- Litter size at birth ranges from 4 to11.

Mali

- Mali is native to Tripura, and is a black colored medium sized pig with pot belly.
- Medium to small bristles are ubiquitously distributed throughout the body.
- Animals are characterized with short erect ears lying perpendicular to body axis and concave snout.
- Adult body weight averages about 68 kg in males and 71 kg in females.
- Average litter size: 5.15 (range 3-7) at birth and 4.46 (range 3-6) at weaning.

Cross bred Pig

T & D/ Jharsuk

- 'JHARSUK' was developed by AICRP on Pig, BAU, Ranchi.
- It has superiority in various economic traits over desi pigs.
- It was developed by crossing Tamworth, a British pig and local one having 50% inheritances of both, thereafter inter-se-mating and by continuous selection for several generations on the basis of black colour, faster growth and better reproductive performances.
- The variety can gain approximately 80 kg body weight at slaughter age of 8-10 months.
- It can produce 8-12 piglets in each farrowing with two farrowing each year.
- This variety has widely been accepted among farmers'.

Rani

- "Rani", the crossbred pig variety has been developed by ICAR-NCR on Pig by crossing Hampshire (exotic breed) with Ghungroo (indigenous breed) to have 50% inheritance of both the breeds.
- The breed characters of "Rani" crossbred has been stabilized for consistent crossbreeding of six generation.
- The breed can gain almost 75 kg body weight at slaughter age of 8 months with 1.98 cm of back fat thickness.

Asha

- "Rani crossbred pig was used to develop Asha cross to have 25% Ghungroo, 25% Hampshire and 50% Duroc inheritance.
- "Asha" can produce 80 kg lean pork at slaughter age of 8 months with 1.75 cm back fat thickness.

HD-K 75

- The All India Coordinated Research project on Pig, Assam Agricultural University at Khanapara, Guwahati has developed HD-K75 variety by systemic crossbreeding and stabilized through 16 generations of inter-se mating with the genetic constitution of 75% Hampshire inheritance and 25% indigenous inheritance of local pigs of Assam.
- The breed can gain almost 74 kg body weight at slaughter age of 8 months with 2.58 cm of back fat thickness.
- The developed variety is found suitable to different agro-climatic conditions of Assam and neighbouring area.
- Litter size at birth: 8-9 piglets
- Weight at 8 months of age: 70-75 kg

Lumasniang

- Lumasniang variety of pig was developed by All India Coordinated Research Project on Pig at ICAR-Research Complex for NEH Region, Barapani by crossing Niang Megha local pig of Meghalaya and Hampshire as exotic breed.
- The variety has better adaptability in hill ecosystem with promising growth rate and feed conservation efficiency, good mothering ability with higher litter size at the time of birth and weaning, good carcass quality and consumer preference in the region.
- Another key feature of the pig variety is suitable to low input tribal production/backyard pig production system.
- The pig variety attained higher body weight of 90-100 kg at 12 months of age, besides higher litter size at weaning as compared to local non-descriptive pigs in the low input tribal production system.
- Litter size at birth: 8-9 piglets
- Weight at 8 months of age: 65-75 kg

Mannuthy White

- Mannuthy White variety was developed under All India Coordinated Research Project on Pig at Kerala Veterinary and Animal Sciences University, Mannuthy, Kerala by crossing pure lines of Large White Yorkshire males with half bred of Large White Yorkshire x Desi females.
- The inheritance level has been stabilized at 75:25 % for LWY and Desi.

- The breed can gain 94 kg bodyweight at slaughter age of 10 months.
- Mannuthy White is well adapted to humid tropical agro-climatic conditions and suited to low input rearing system of Kerala.
- The developed variety is useful for mitigating demand of improved pig germplasm of the state of Kerala and adjoining areas.
- Litter size at birth: 9-10 piglets
- Weight at 8 months of age: 75-80 kg

TANUVAS KPM Gold

- The crossbred pig variety "TANUVAS KPM Gold" was developed by AICRP on Pig at PGRIAS, Kattupakkam The crossbred pig variety was devolved by crossing Large White Yorkshire with Desi pig of Tamil Nadu.
- The inheritance level has been stabilized at 75:25 % for LWY and Desi.
- The developed variety is adapted to local climatic condition of the state with litter size at birth of 8-9 and average body weight of 72 kg at 8 months.

SVVU T-17

- The crossbred pig variety SVVU T-17 was developed by AICRP on Pig centre of Sri Venkateswara Veterinary University (SVVU), Tirupati.
- The variety was developed by crossing of Large White Yorkshire with Desi pig of the state with 75% exotic inheritance.
- The developed crossbred pig variety can attain 85.48 kg body weight at slaughter age of 10 months with 8.1 litter size at birth.
- Litter size at birth: 8-9 piglets
- Weight at 8 months of age: 70-75 kg

Landlly

- Landlly variety was developed under All India Coordinated Research Project on Pig at ICAR-Indian Veterinary Research Institute, Bareilly by crossing pure lines of Landrace males with Gurrah females.
- The inheritance level has been stabilized at 75:25 % for Landrace and Gurrah.
- The breed can gain 75-80 kg body weight at slaughter age of 8 months.
- The variety is well adapted to hot humid tropical agro-climatic conditions.
- Litter size at birth: 7-8 piglets

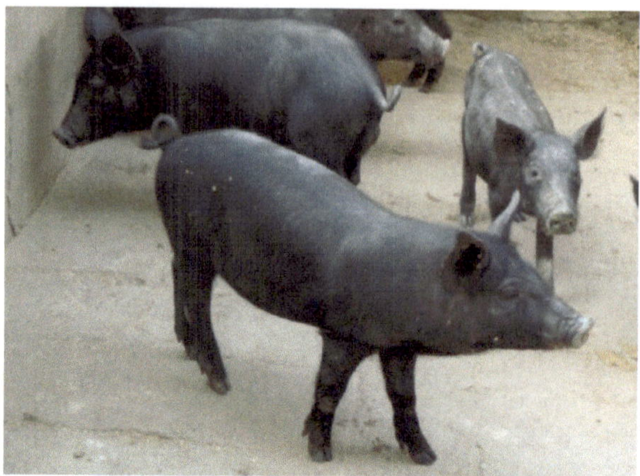

Figure 1: T & D pig

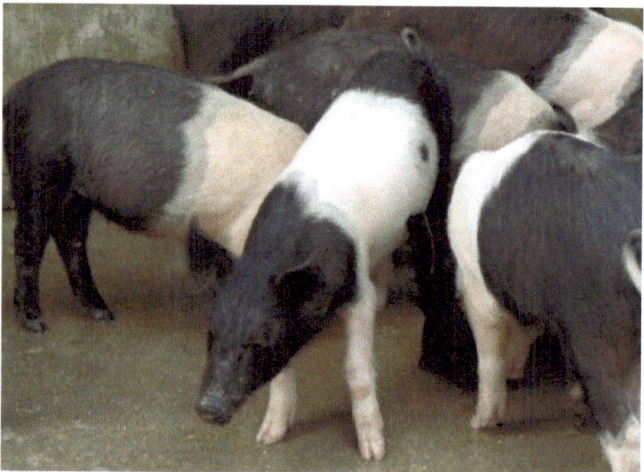

Figure 2: Hampshire pig

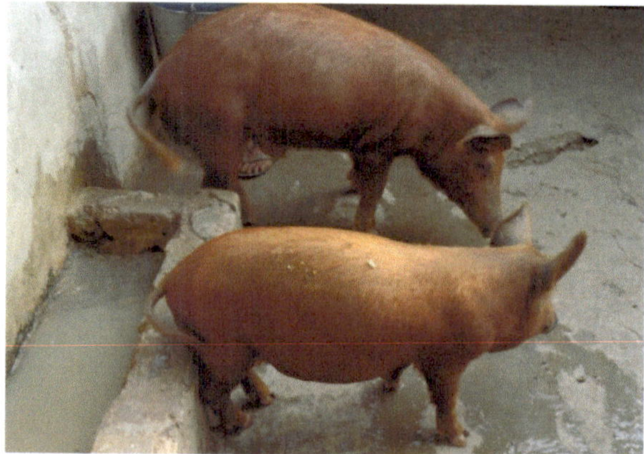

Figure 3: Tamworth pig

4

Pig Reproductive System

Successful management strategies require an understanding of the pig reproductive system. Profitability in pig production farm is primarily limited by reproductive efficiency. Increasing reproductive efficiency lowers the cost of each pig sold. Increased pig marketing per female could reduce the number of sows required or increase the overall number of pigs marketed per year. Nonetheless, improving reproductive performance requires time. There are no quick fixes for enhancing reproductive performance. To improve the reproductive parameters of swine farms, sound management approaches and a rigorous genetic selection programme are required.

Sow's Reproductive Organ

Understanding the reproductive system of the sow is required for a successful mating programme, whether AI or natural service is used. The ovaries are the principal structures of the female reproductive tract, and they serve two functions:

1. To produce ova, the female germ cells and
2. To produce the hormones progesterone and estrogen.

- Each ovary is enclosed by a thin membrane called the infundibulum, which serves as a funnel for eggs to be collected and directed to the oviduct. The oviduct, which is 6-10 inches long, serves as the site of fertilisation.
- The uterus has two horns. Each is about 2-3 feet long. They are the site of foetal development and serve as a channel for sperm to reach the oviduct. The uterine body is placed at the confluence of the two uterine horns and is small in comparison to other species.
- The cervix is the muscle junction between the vagina and the uterus. It is the location of sperm depositing. It dilates during heat but contracts throughout the rest of the estrous cycle and throughout pregnancy.
- The vagina extends from the cervix to the vulva and serves as a channel for urine and piglets during delivery.

- The vulva is the reproductive tract's outermost section. It commonly turns red and swollen soon before estrus, and this swelling is usually more noticeable in gilts than in sows.
- The hypothalamus, located at the base of the brain, secretes gonadotropin releasing hormone (GnRH), which directs the anterior pituitary gland to secrete FSH and LH into the blood, stimulating the production of the ovarian hormones, oestrogen and progesterone, which control the reproductive process. The posterior pituitary gland secretes oxytocin.

Puberty in sow

- Around 5 months of age, the sow is ready to reproduce and shows signs of being in heat. Certain slow-growing animals and underfed animals will be older when they reach puberty.
- When the pig initially reaches puberty, gilt should not be utilised for breeding. It is better to let her mature for another month before breeding her. She will then be more capable of carrying and suckling a large litter of kids.
- If the sow is not mated, she will go into heat every three weeks for the rest of the year.
- Most pig breeds reach puberty about 5 months of age, although some, such as the Chinese pig, come into heat for the first time at 3 months of age if they have access to adequate nutrition and water.
- Only sows with 14 teats should be utilised for breeding to ensure that her entire litter is fed.

Estrous cycle

- Estrus is displayed on a regular basis throughout the year by non-pregnant and non-lactating sows or gilts.
- The estrous cycle is usually 21 days long and is defined as the interval between the onsets of one estrus and the onset of the next. The cycle length might range between 18 and 24 days.
- Breastfeeding hinders the estrous cycle, and sows will not return to heat until the litter is weaned.
- The number of days between weaning and estrus is regulated by factors like as lactation length, parity, season, and nutritional level, but should be between 4 and 7 days.
- The onset and termination of estrus, as well as estrus behaviour, are consistent, with individual variances amongst females.

- The primary and most reliable indicator of estrus is “standing” while another sow or boar mounts.
- When the herd-person applies the “back pressure test,” many females will stand.
- A higher proportion of females will respond to the “back pressure test” if a boar is present.
- As a result, employing an intact or vasectomized boar is an essential aspect of a routine heat detection programme.
- Boars generate pheromones in their salivary glands, which trigger the female’s standing reflex; mature boars outperform juvenile boars in activating this response.

Secondary signs of estrus include

- Red, swollen vulva which is usually more pronounced in gilts than in sows.
- Increased nervous activity.
- Desire to seek the boar.
- Loss of appetite.
- Male-like sexual behavior (pursuing, nosing and mounting other females).
- Change in vocalization (grunts and growls).
- Increase in vaginal mucous

Ovulation

- As estrus or heat approaches, each ovary develops 6-10 follicles or “blister-like” structures.
- Follicular growth accelerates roughly three days before estrus and is affected by FSH, or follicle stimulating hormone, which is secreted by the pituitary gland.
- Each follicle contains a maturing ovum. Granulosa cells within the follicle secrete oestrogen, a hormone responsible for the usual symptoms of estrus.
- LH stimulates ovulation, or the release of the ova. Ovulation happens approximately 40 hours following the commencement of estrus.
- Estrus or heat can persist as little as 12 hours in gilts and as much as 60 hours or more in sows. Because the precise start of estrus is rarely known, it is suggested that a female accept at least two matings during estrus. This ensures that sperm are available at the optimal time relative to ovulation for fertilisation to take place.

- Inseminate a female 12 hours after the onset of standing estrus is noted, and then again 18 to 24 hours later. The optimal time to mate will differ amongst farms. Two services, as opposed to one, may enhance conception rate and litter size by 10%.
- The follicular structures are converted into corpora lutea after ovulation. From about day 1 to 2 after mating, they produce and release the hormone progesterone, which is responsible for pregnancy maintenance.
- If pregnancy does not occur, the uterus secretes prostaglandin, forcing the corpora lutea to revert and stop generating progesterone around day 17 of the cycle. A fresh set of follicles begins to grow at this point, and the operation is repeated. If conception occurs, the corpora lutea remains functioning and continues to release progesterone throughout the pregnancy.

Several factors can influence ovulation rate or number of ova shed.

1. **Age.** Sows may ovulate 18-20 ova while gilts may ovulate 12-14 ova.
2. **Nutrition.** Flushing may amplify ovulation rate yet may have little effect on the ultimate litter size.
3. **Breed.** Crossbred females usually have a higher ovulation rate than either of the parent breeds.

Fertilization, Embryonic and Fetal Development

- During mating or insemination, sperm is deposited in the cervix.
- The boar deposits thirty to sixty billion sperm during mating or two to six billion during insemination, but only a small part of them reach the oviduct and the location of the ova.
- Uterine contractions cause sperm transfer. The pituitary gland's production of oxytocin stimulates these contractions. Its discharge is mediated by mating-related cues. Tactile stimulation during and after insemination, as well as close touch with a boar, may increase sperm transfer.
- Sperm must be present in the female for 6-10 hours before it may fertilise. This is known as capacitation, and it involves both physical and physiological changes within the sperm.
- Fertilization takes place in the upper third of the oviduct. If the female is mated to a fertile boar at the correct time relative to ovulation, the fertility rate is around 100%.

- The blastocysts enter the uterus about 2 days after fertilisation. They are in the 4-8 cell stage and begin to space themselves equally in the uterine horns. During this stage, blastocysts can move from one horn to another.

Gestation period

- Fetal growth occurs between the attachment of fertilised embryos to the uterus and the day before farrowing. Piglets develop and grow within the sow during the gestation period. The gestation period is around 115 days.
- One of the most important stages of pregnancy occurs between days 11 and 16 following mating. The blastocysts grow into long, stringy masses that begin to link to the uterine wall. Because of attachment failures, the largest probable loss in litter size may occur during this stage of development.
- On average, 17 ova are shed during estrus, but only around 12 are counted as blastocysts after the connection is established. There are some theories as to why the number of blastocysts that can link in a given uterus is limited.
- Embryonic survival may be linked to specific uterine secretions. Environmental stressors including high temperatures and struggle as a result of mixing or regrouping animals also have a negative impact on implantation and embryo survival. In order for a pregnancy to continue, at least four blastocysts must be present.
- Embryos that die before the age of 35-40 are usually reabsorbed by the dam. However, from day 36 onwards, gradual calcification of the bones occurs, and fatalities occurring after this point result in mummification.
- From conception through farrowing, the average gestation period is 115 days. Throughout gestation, the piglet develops from a microscopic sperm and ovum union into a fully grown individual weighing 3 to 3.5 pounds.

Mothering instinct

- A female domestic pig usually gives birth to 10-14 piglets after around 115 days. The sow exhibits impatience and a considerable tendency to squirt three to four days before the delivery. In free-range systems, the sow departs the group and seeks her own location to build a litter nest. Other pigs are no longer permitted, and the sow is violently attacking them.
- Pregnant sows, standing on slatted floors, have no nesting material available. The animals consequently show a number of behavioural disorders such as the stereotypical “empty digging” or “bar biting”. The agitation of the sows is reduced when straw is offered as bedding.

- The farrowing takes about three to four hours. The very superior piglets are born with open eyes and can run just a few minutes after birth.
- Immediately after delivery, the sow leaves the nest for a brief period of time to defecate and urinate. If she is not allowed to do so, as in the crate, she frequently holds the defecation for so long that it causes a blockage.
- A suckling order forms immediately after birth, with the stronger piglets occupying the front teats of the sow and the weaker piglets occupying the back teats. The piglets spend the first week in the nest together. They leave the nest for the first time in the second week to explore the surroundings and play with the other animals in the group.

Reproduction after farrowing

- The number of pigs sold per sow each year drives pig production system productivity and is determined by farrowing frequency. The proclivity of sows to remain anovulatory when suckling a litter may be the principal constraint to farrowing frequency and, thus, reproductive effectiveness of sow breeding herds.
- Upon weaning, the majority of sows resumes oestrous cycling and ovulates swiftly and synchronously, which simplifies insemination management, animal housing, and feeding; allows animals to be managed in batches; and aids in environmental and disease control. Lactation anoestrus, on the other hand, limits the flexibility with which pig production systems can be adapted to satisfy the changing needs of the producer, customer, retailer, and government organisations, as well as the needs of the piglet and sow.
- Weaning is now dictated by the requirement to maximise farrowing frequency while minimising successive litter size. Weaning is typically performed in commercial settings at 3-4 weeks of age, resulting in significant stress, which reduces post-weaning piglet feed intake, growth, and survival, and hence reduces production efficiency. But advancing the weaning age to 5 to 7 weeks can reduce piglet stress and increase post-weaning performance and survival. This delay reduces the amount of litters produced per sow per year, making the alteration unsustainable.
- Selection for larger litter numbers could protect breeding herd efficiency from the unfavourable effects of higher weaning age. Larger litter numbers, on the other hand, result in lower mean birth weights, which can have a negative impact on piglet performance and survival as well as production efficiencies.
- Bigger litters are also associated with longer parturitions, higher peri- and pre-weaning mortality, and slower growth to weaning, higher labour

and intervention expenditures, and an increase in the number of days to slaughter weight. Therefore, lower-birth-weight piglets are more likely to benefit from later weaning ages, effectively establishing a vicious cycle in which the need to delay weaning is greater. As a result, the question of whether constant selection for increasing litter size is economically sustainable is raised.

Synchronization of estrous

- The best reproductive performance of the breeding herd is critical for profitable pig farming and the success of artificial insemination programmes. The reproductive cycle of the female breeding herd dominates the calendar in piggery units. Successive pig production will deteriorate if sufficient female breeding herds are not available for subsequent breeding. Female reproduction management for estrus induction and synchronisation is thus regarded as an important reproductive management method for increasing pig reproductive performance.
- It is ideal for pig farmers to have synchronised estrus occurring at an early stage and at the same time for a group of animals so that they can be bred at the same time and deliver offspring at the same time. The juveniles will grow into a group of pigs of roughly same age that can be handled with the same feed housing and marketing. The application of appropriate and cost-effective strategies for estrus induction and synchronised breeding in replacement gilts and weaned sows that do not return to estrus when predicted can improve reproductive performance. Additionally, estrus synchronisation can help with fixed-time insemination, which is a highly effective method of getting pregnant.
- There are numerous hormonal-agent-based strategies for pig estrus induction and synchronisation. The bulk of ovarian activity control approaches focus on managing events that lead to follicular maturation and ovulation or modifying the luteal phase.
- Prior to implementing a certain approach, it is critical to clearly grasp the estrous cycle of pigs. The estrous cycle has a normal duration of 21 days and is made up of a somewhat prolonged luteal phase (approximately 16 days) and a shorter follicular phase (roughly 5 days). During the luteal phase, corpora lutea-containing ovaries release progesterone, which regulates follicular development to the medium-sized follicle stage and thereby prevents the beginning of estrus. At about 12–14 days of the luteal phase, uterine release of prostaglandin F2α causes regression of corpora lutea and therefore progesterone level decreases.

- Clearing the progesterone blockage permits the pituitary gonadotropins, luteinizing hormone and follicle stimulating hormone, to resume secretory patterns, allowing follicular development to be completed with oestrogen production and the commencement of behavioural estrus.
- Throughout the last few decades, research has been conducted to create and validate a range of procedures for regulating estrus and ovarian activity in pigs using exogenous hormone preparations, primarily to delay follicle growth, control follicle development, or induce ovulation.

Male reproductive organ

- The boar has large ecliptical testes with wide testicular tunics and adjacent massive epididymides that are connected to the testis by efferent ducts and the urethra via the ductus deferens.
- The epididymis tail is positioned dorsally inside the scrotum. The boar epididymis is divided into separate regions: the beginning segment, caput, corpus, and cauda epididymis.
- A scrotal raphe divides the scrotum into two halves when it is in the sub-anal position. The testis descends shortly before delivery.
- The boar's seminiferous tubules are exceptionally tightly packed, resulting in thick parenchyma.
- In the boar, the vesicular gland and bulbourethral glands are enormous and provide the mass of seminal plasma volume.
- The prostate gland is unusually tiny. A pig's penis is long and fibroelastic, with a sigmoid flexure and a spiralling tip lying within a two-compartment prepuce. Its anatomy facilitates cervical penetration and intracervical sperm deposition while mating with a sow.
- Once a boar reaches puberty, waves of spermatozoa begin to form every 3-4 days, taking 5-6 weeks to reach fertilizational potential. This practise should continue indefinitely as long as boars are collected, which is normally until they are 20-24 months old.

5

Artificial Insemination In Pig

Successful artificial insemination (AI) is necessary to maximise productivity on any pig farm. There are two types of breeding methods viz. natural mating and artificial insemination. Natural mating involves mating with a boar of superior breed qualities. On the field, only a few farmers have their own boar, and they are employed without regard for genetic merit, breed, or superiority of boar. Only the best quality breeding boar available in the area should be used to produce better piglets with larger litter sizes. Artificial insemination involves artificially collecting sperm from a proven boar, evaluating it for perfection, and depositing it into the cervix of a receptive sow. Artificial means are used for both collection and insemination. This expertise offers an extraordinary opportunity for the genetic upgrading of the animal species to which it is applied. Furthermore, it provides the most cost-effective approach of preserving genetic diversity in a population.

Collection of semen, dilution and processing

- Despite the development of mechanised semen collection techniques, semen is frequently collected by gloved hand from a boar trained to mount a dummy sow. Dummy sows should be well-built, with no sharp edges, and placed in a semen collection room with a non-slippery floor.
- The end of the penis is tightly gripped with a gloved hand, and the collection operation begins with hard pressure to the spiral end of the penis with the hand, preventing the penis from rotating. This process simulates the pressure exerted by the sow's vagina's corkscrew curvature. Polyvinyl gloves can be used to collect sperm.
- The first part of the ejaculate should be thrown away. It is a clear, watery fluid devoid of sperm. It is necessary to collect the sperm-rich part. It has a chalky look and comprises 80-90% of all sperm cells found in ejaculate.
- Once the sperm-rich fraction is finished, the remaining ejaculate is a clearer, watery fluid that should not be collected.
- The ejaculation can last up to 5 to 8 minutes, but it might last up to 15 minutes. Semen is collected in quantities ranging from 100 to 300 ml.

- The sperm should be extended within 15 minutes of being collected. The process should be carried out in a warm room with sanitary and sterile equipment. The extender is mixed into the sperm, and cold shock should be avoided by gradually lowering the temperature.
- Semen collection from boars occurs generally twice each week at AI-centres.
- A typical ejaculate contains enough sperm to inseminate 15 to 25 sows using conventional AI.
- In 80-100 ml, each dose should include 2-3 billion spermatozoa sperms.

Different AI methods

Artificial insemination is the introduction and release of sperm into a gilt's or sow's reproductive canal. The most common form of AI is to send sperm to the cervix (trans-cervical AI); however, firms have developed catheters and ways to transfer sperm deeper into the reproductive system:

- Post-cervical AI allows for a decrease in spermatozoa (sperm cells) in the semen to one third of those required for standard AI
- Deep-intrauterine AI allows for a decrease in spermatozoa (sperm cells) by 5–20 times less than standard AI

All changes to AI procedure should be done with the approval of the genetics expert that provides the sperm dosages, the farm veterinarian, and the AI staff. It is critical to give frequent staff training on both new AI techniques and standard agricultural techniques.

Benefits of AI

There are numerous benefits, but the most important ones are listed below:

- It allows for the widespread utilisation of better male germplasm to produce genetically improved offspring.
- It makes it easier to use and transport sperm over long distances.
- It reduces the risk of sexually transmitted infections.
- It makes the introduction of new genetic material easier.
- It also minimises the spread of infectious diseases such as Swine Fever and Foot and Mouth Disease.
- Al has a wide range of applications in the creation of rotational or terminal crossbreeding programmes.

Important points for successful AI

- Time and approach are two critical aspects in AI's rapid adoption.
- Strict sanitary precautions should be implemented when handling sperm and during insemination.
- Clean the vulva to remove filth that could clog the catheter head.
- For each sow, always use a new/sterile catheter.
- Rough handling, temperature shock, and light exposure all degrade sperm quality.
- Supply of high-quality pig sperm
- Accurate ways for detecting estrus or heat in the breeding sow, as well as a method of inseminating the sperm into the reproductive tract of the receptive female.
- Ascertain that the sow or gilt is in a standing heat.
- The catheter head is placed into the vulva with considerable anti-clockwise twisting and gently pushed forward and upwards at a 45-degree angle into the reproductive tract.
- When resistance is detected, the catheter is pushed slightly back to achieve a firm lock. Once the catheter is securely in place, the semen bag is attached to it and lifted above the level of the vulva. The uterine contractions will draw the sperm from the bag and into the uterine tract.
- Moderate squeezing pressure can also be used to ensure proper and uniform semen flow. Continue to stimulate the animal by massaging her flanks and putting weight on her back.
- After insemination, extract the catheter by rotating it clockwise.

Post AI care

- The catheter is remained in the sow for 5 minutes in order to sustain cervical stimulation and uterine contractions.
- To prevent backflow of semen, the catheter should be doubled over and bound at the conclusion of semen intake.
- 12 and 24 hours after the last insemination, check the animal for standing heat.
- She should quit standing within 12 hours of insemination.
- Dates of A.I., 21-day check-due date, boar ID, and any events such as bleeding or other observations should be recorded.
- Frequent estrus detection and pregnancy diagnosis are recommended to assess conception and pregnancy.

Timing of AI

Exact estrus identification is required for accurate timing. Before ovulation may occur, viable sperm must be present in the sow's uterus. Oocytes have a short lifetime of roughly 8 hours after ovulation. Sperm cells survive in the sow's reproductive tract for about 24 hours. Ovulation timing varies between individuals, breeds, and age groups. Ovulation is thought to occur roughly 66-75% of the time during standing estrus.

The following table depicts the general timing of AI for Gilts and sows:

Groups	Single AI after detected estrus	Double AI after first detected estrus/heat
Gilts	24 – 30 hrs (10-14 hrs after Standing heat)	1st AI: 10-14 hrs (6 hrs after Standing heat) 2nd AI: 12 hrs-after 1st AI
Sows	28 – 36 hrs (12-16 hrs after Standing heat)	1st AI: 12-16 hrs (6-8 hrs after Standing heat) 2nd AI: 12 hrs-after 1st AI

6

Reproduction Management on Pig Farm

To achieve maximum reproductive efficiency, animals recently introduced into the breeding herd should be closely monitored. Effective management results in an increase in the number of live farrowed and weaned pigs. The following boar management strategies will aid in increasing fertility.

Care and Management of Breeding Boar

- Boars should be fed at a level of energy that prevents excessive fat deposition. This approach should ensure that they are physically fit and sexually active.
- To fulfil the minimum daily recommended amount, nutrients other than energy need be delivered.
- Boars must be at least 7.5 months old and to be tested for reproductive health.
- The examination should be finished before the mating season begins so that problem boars can be identified and removed.

Boars should be evaluated on the following criteria.

- **Libido:** Observe the boar's ferociousness and desire to mate. Boars may need help through at least one mating experience.
- **Mounting:** Boars must have the capability to mount properly. Some boars may be interested in mounting but lameness, arthritis, or injury may stop them.
- **Mating:** Observe the boar's capability to erect the penis and correctly enter the gilt. Scrutinize the boar's penis for normal size and condition. Penis abnormalities encountered sporadically are: (1) adhered penis, (2) limp penis, (3) infantile penis, and (4) coiling of the penis in the diverticulum. Boars showing these problems should not be used to produce breeding stock.

- **Semen:** A few boars do not produce sperm cells. As a result, the sperm of young boars should be tested. Allowing a boar to mount gilt in standing heat is the simplest way to gather semen from a boar. Put a rubber glove on one hand and, once the pig begins to grow his penis, grab the corkscrew end of his penis securely and slowly bring the penis ahead once extended ejaculation begins. Collect the entire ejaculate carefully. A new boar's first ejaculate may not be a precise test and should not be utilised for evaluation.
- **Test Mating:** To complete the soundness evaluation, two or three gilts should be bred and cautiously checked as to whether they return to estrus within 4 weeks.

Care and Management of Breeding Sow

- To avoid overweight circumstances, gilts' energy intake should be limited.
- To satisfy the minimum daily suggested amounts, nutrients other than energy need be delivered.
- Transferring gilts to different pens, increasing exercise, and daily exposure to boars will assist encourage the start of estrus between 160 and 180 days of age.
- To maximise the chances of big litters and to avoid dystocia, breeding should be delayed until the second or third estrus of gilt.
- Gilts that do not conceive after two estrous phases of mating should be culled. Similarly, gilts that have not displayed heat by 9 months of age should also be culled.
- Throughout gestation, gilts should be fed appropriately so that they do not become overly fat.

General signs of heat

Early heat signs

- General impatience
- Vulva turns red and is swollen
- White mucus discharge

Service/AI period signs

- Vulva becomes less red and swollen
- Slimy mucus discharge
- Propensity to mount and be mounted by others.
- The sow or gilt will stand still when pressure is applied to her back.

Post oestrus-period signs

- The sow/gilt will not stand still when pressure is applied to her back.
- The swelling of the vulva disappears.

How to induce heat

A sow may not come into heat in time after farrowing. Farmers should utilise the following strategies to induce heat:

- For 3-5 days, spray the sow's or gilt's pen with boar urine every morning.
- 1 kg fresh or dried lotus (Semen nelumbinis) seeds, crushed. Combine it with 20 kg dry feed. Give it twice a day to the sow for 5-7 days.
- Put the sow in the same pen as the boar.
- Bring the sow close to the boar every day when the heat is expected.
- Before feeding, put the sow and boar together.
- Give the sow/gilt 1 - 2 kg of extra feed every day for 10 days before service. This should also be done for a week after service.
- Provide 0.5 kg more feed per day during the last month of pregnancy, but progressively reduce this one week before farrowing.

Minimum Breeding Ages for Boars and Gilts

The minimum age for successful breeding in boars is 7.5 months. Gilts should be bred on the second or third heat to take advantage of the expected increase in ovulation rate that usually occurs following puberty.

Age to breed gilts	8 months
Age to breed boars	7.5 month
Weight of breeding gilts	100-120 kg
Length of heat period	2-3 days
Occurrence of heat after weaning	2-10 days

Induced Farrowing in sow

Farrowing can be a stressful course for both pig caretaker and sow involved. The procedure of induction alleviates part of the stress by allowing the caretaker to handle the sow and piglets correctly during farrowing hours. The key strategy to reduce piglet mortality around farrowing is through management and the ability to provide timely support. Proper use of induction can increase the likelihood that the caretaker will be accessible when farrowing occurs.

Before considering induction on the farm, farmers should talk with their veterinarian to learn more about induction methodology. On many swine farms, prostaglandin and oxytocin are used to induce farrowing. Prostaglandin is the most commonly used inducer during farrowing, and oxytocin is used in addition to prostaglandin if necessary.

Prostaglandin

The sow naturally produces prostaglandin to end the pregnancy and begin the farrowing process. Exogenous prostaglandins allow the caretaker to synchronise farrowing across multiple sows or to a preferred time of day for attendance considerations. For the effectiveness of prostaglandin and the safety of the sow and piglets, the timing of prostaglandin usage should be chosen based on the projected farrowing dates. Most farms employ a prostaglandin injection on day 114 of gestation, allowing sows with shorter gestation durations to farrow naturally and sows with longer gestation periods to farrow somewhat earlier. On days 112-114, using prostaglandin had no negative effects and minimises variation in farrowing timing across a group of sows. The use of prostaglandins on or before day 111 is considered early. Farrowing typically begins 12-24 hours after the injection of prostaglandin. Prostaglandin induction, when administered correctly and in cooperation with a veterinarian, can reduce the occurrence of stillbirth piglets and improve live-born survival rates due to the benefits of caretaker attendance at farrowing.

Oxytocin

The administration of oxytocin exogenously promotes uterine contractions. The primary purpose of using oxytocin is to shorten the farrowing duration and the intervals between each piglet's birth. Although oxytocin can be administered without first employing prostaglandin, it should only be utilised when the cervix has been thoroughly dilated. It is important to note that whereas prostaglandin induces parturition, oxytocin mostly aids in the farrowing process once parturition has begun.

The timing of oxytocin administration is critical. During the farrowing process, oxytocin is typically employed. When used in conjunction with prostaglandin, oxytocin can be administered as early as 20-24 hours after the prostaglandin has been administered. Nonetheless, it is essential to see a veterinarian and keep in mind that dilatation may not have occurred by this point. While adopting a synchronisation protocol, gilts are less predictable in terms of farrowing timing. The use of oxytocin should be limited; in most situations, it is recommended to limit the use of oxytocin to two doses each sow. When utilising oxytocin to aid in farrowing, it is important to be strategic and cautious.

Consult with a veterinarian before utilising any medications on your sows, especially oxytocin. Misuse of oxytocin can result in an increase in dystocia during farrowing. This may also increase the number of stillbirths. Working on an induction plan with your veterinarian can help reduce these concerns.

7
Attainable Performance Goals in Pig Farming

Different economis characters of pig have been discussed in the following table.

Economic character	**Excellent**	**Good**	**Poor**	**Goal**
Pregnancy rate				
Gilt	>80%	70-80%	<70%	90%
Sow	>90%	80-90%	<80%	95%
Farrowing rate				
Gilt	>80%	70-80%	<70%	85%
Sow	>90%	80-90%	<80%	95%
Litter size at birth				
Gilt	>09	7-8	<7	10
Sow	>10	8-9	<8	11
Still birth at birth	<0.8	0.8-1.5	>1.5	0.5
Av. Piglet weight at birth	>1.5	1.25-1.5	<1.25	1.5
Litter size after 56 days of birth				
Gilt	>8	6.5-7.5	<6.5	9
Sow	>9	7.5-8.5	<7.5	10
Weaning wt	> 12 kg	9-11 kg	<9kg	14 kg
Av weight gain till 10 month	> 0.5 kg	0.3-0.4 kg	<0.3 kg	0.5 kg
No. of Farrowing per year	>2	1.6-2.0	>1.6	2.2
No. of piglets weaned per year per sow	>16	12-15	<12	18
Feed conversion ability	<2.75:1	2.75-3.25:1	>3.25:1	2.5:1

Economic character	Excellent	Good	Poor	Goal
Mortality Rate				
0-2 month	<10%	10-12%	>12%	<10%
2-10 month	<2%	3-5%	>5%	<2%
Sow	<2%	3-4%	>4%	<2%

8

Breeding Management

Pigs are inherently prolific, and two farrowings per year under optimal management conditions should be planned. One boar must be kept for every ten sows for optimal fertility. Breed the animals at their most active heat cycle (12 to 24 hours of heat). After every 21 days, the sows come into heat. Proper feeding and handling promotes heat, which facilitates breeding and results in larger litter numbers. In addition to grains, there is fish meal, skim milk or butter milk feed can be administered 2-3 weeks before breeding to allow for a 200-300 gm/day increase in body weight. The normal gestation period for a sow is 112-115 days, and the usual litter size is 8-10 piglets. Larger litters with higher birth weights are produced by older sows.

Care and management of boar

The boar should be confined to its own enclosure. They should not be overfed or underfed because both will impair their ability to reproduce. It should be meaty, thrifty, and not too fatty. The feed requirements cover both maintenance and reproduction. During the off-season, the boar should be given a lot of grass and legume hay, along with 2kg of concentrate mixture. Two weeks before breeding season, an extra 0.5 kg of concentrate may be provided.

Boars should not be used for breeding until they are 8 months old. In a season, a young boar can handle 15-20 sows, whereas an experienced boar may handle 25-45 sows. A boar can be permitted to serve before being fed. During the breeding season, just one service is permitted each day. Older sows may be used during the breeding season. Elderly sows can be used to mate with younger boars.

The boar should have unrestricted access to water, and the boar pen should be kept clean and dry. It is preferable to avoid moisture. On a daily basis, the boar should be cleansed, rinsed, and maintained clean. Boar lameness can be avoided by regularly trimming their hoof. Bolt cutters can be used to remove boar tusks, thereby protecting sows and attendants.

Newly purchased boars should be housed separately for 2-3 weeks to limit the possibility of disease introduction into the farm.

The reproductive performance of a herd boar is contingent on proper care and management. Boars are frequently ignored, especially newly purchased boars on the journey and after they reach home. There are important steps in herd boar care and management that will help eliminate sources of difficulty.

Care in transporting the boar

- Provide sufficient loading and unloading facilities.
- Ascertain that the truck has been cleaned and disinfected.
- Offer suitable bedding
- Protect against wind, harsh cold, rain, snow, and heat.
- Transporting boars that are unfamiliar with each other or feeding intensively before transit, especially in hot weather, is not recommended.
- When you receive the breeding boar, quarantine them.

The new boar should be housed in comfortable conditions away from other animals and clear of drainage from other lots. The following steps should be taken:

- Clean and sanitise the sheds (quarters) a few weeks before bringing the new boar.
- Do not mix boars that have never met before.
- Give a dry, and well-ventilated sleeping area of 15-20 square feet.
- Examine whether the quarters give shelter from inclement weather.
- Place the boar away from a gilt pen.
- Give appropriate shade; if natural shade is not available, at least 30 square feet of artificial shade should be provided.
- Give a large enough exercise space – at least 1/4 acre; preferably legume pasture. Outside exercise area for all over year is one of the most important criteria for keeping the pig virile and thrifty.
- To encourage activity, create distinct feeding and sleeping areas. This typically stimulates exercise and competitiveness during meal time, encouraging the pig to start eating.
- Separate the newly purchased boar from the herd for at least 30 days in a containment.

Feeding to grow or maintain the herd boar

- Few farm meals are nutrient-deficient responsible for disrupting a boar's reproductive function. A boar, on the other hand, may become permanently or temporarily sterile if a nutrient-deficient diet is provided for an extended period of time.
- Most breeders tend to over-feed their boars. This is a wasteful that contributes to overeating, decreased libido, and sluggishness.

Handling boars before and after breeding season

In breeding seasons, only boars of the same age and size are run together, as long as they are placed together at a young age and their teeth are frequently cut. Teeth should be removed from elder boars each year, or as needed, before breeding season. Bolt cutters, hoof trimmers, or a hack saw can be used to do this work. Occasionally mature boars are known to become furious and attack.

Managing the breeding animals requires patience and good judgement, as harsh treatment might cause old boars to become violent or young boars to become too shy to mate.

Health check and care

The majority of health problems can be avoided by buying boars from herds that appear to be disease and parasite free. This is usually determined before purchasing a boar by carefully observing the herd.

After bringing the pig to farm, keep them isolated for as long as possible - 4 to 5 weeks is best. Veterinarian is critical to the health of boar and herd.

The following are health recommendation for breeders:

- A negative brucellosis test and leptospirosis immunisation are required before acquiring a boar.
- Check to see if the boar has received an erysipelas vaccination.
- If the owner has not recently treated for internal and external parasites, do so.
- Keep a close eye on the boar during the isolation period for signs of illness, sluggishness, or coughing. Contact your veterinarian if his temperature rises beyond 103 degree Fahrenheit.
- Three to four weeks after bringing boars farm, do a brucellosis and leptospirosis blood test. This is a precautionary measure to guarantee that they did not contract one of these diseases before to purchasing or while on his route to farm. Veterinarian should thoroughly examine while they are in isolation.

- If the boar becomes ill and develops a fever, refrain from using them for 8 to 10 weeks after the fever has disappeared.
- Be certain that the sanitation and health programme is of the greatest standard.
- Stop all antibiotics from the feed three weeks after arriving for one month before breeding.
- Three weeks before breeding and three weeks after isolation, rotate the new boar through the sow lot. Let the new boar to run with bred sows or in lots used by sows to be bred to boar before breeding to expose boar to herd health issues.

Important Managemental Practices

- Proper feeding is essential before and throughout the breeding season. A boar's performance is typically poor when effective management methods are not followed.
- Condition the boar by increasing meals to 3 kg, six to eight weeks before breeding season.
- A fertility test should be performed at least 30 days before using the boar. Manual mating to five or six healthy gilts about to be culled is one of the most efficient approaches. If more over one-third of these gilts go into heat within 28 days of mating, the fertility of the boar may be called into question. Boars should be evaluated by someone who has had sufficient training in evaluating boars.

The following parameters should be included in the evaluation

- The reproductive organs' anatomy and development are investigated.
- A test of the ability to achieve a normal erection, followed by a normal penis extension and acceptable service performance.
- Sperm motility, concentration, and morphological and anatomical anomalies are all evaluated.
- When the temperature rises, hand mating should be done early in the morning and/or late in the evening. Feed the boar once a day, preferably after it has been used.
- The sow should be bred at least twice during the heat cycle, ideally on the latter day of the first day and early on the second day. Two services, according to studies, boost conception by 30% on the first heat and litter size by one pig.

- Because individual boars vary in desire, aggressiveness, and ability to serve, calculating the proper breeding load for boars is difficult.

Table Recommended breeding age and service of boars with different systems of mating

Age in months	Pasture mating	Hand mating
7 or less	None	None
7 to 9	6 to 8 in 21 days	10 to 15 in 21 days
9 to 12	8 to 10 in 21 days	15 to 20 in 21 days
12 to 18	10 to 12 in 21 days	20 to 25 in 21 days
18 or over	12 to 15 in 21 days	25 to 30 in 21 days

Breeding procedure

- Hand mating is more common in swine than it is in cattle or sheep. In reality, it is practically prevalent in purebred swine herds, and some commercial producers use the same method.
- A breeding crate is indicated when a mature, heavy boar is to be bred to gilts or when a boar pig is to be bred to large. Animals that have been naturally reproducing may refuse to utilise a box or may reproduce reluctantly. If a breeding crate is not available, two hay bales placed one on each side of gilt may suffice as a substitute.

Two strategies are proposed for field mating with commercial herds:

- Divide the herd and have one boar per group
- Alternate boars in the herd; that is, use one boar or set of boars one day and another boar or set of boars the next day.

During summer months, you can get best conception rates by allowing the boars in breeding pens from sundown to sunup.

Age of breeding stock

When well-developed gilts are 8-9 months old, they can be bred to farrow. Growth and development, rather than age, determines breeding efficiency of gilt or sow. Gilts should weigh at least 100 kg before breeding. The oestrous phase (up to the fifth) increases the rate of ovulation after puberty. Deferring breeding gilts until the second or third oestrous cycle is advantageous. In consecutive pregnancies, litter size increases on average until the fifth or sixth litter. After her fifth or sixth litter, it is recommended to cull the sow from a breeding herd or a commercial herd since the litter size drops.

9

Mating System in Pig

Pure-breeding

Mating purebred individuals of the same breed. The progeny share the same genetic make-up. The primary goal of pure-breeding is to identify and propagate superior genes for use in commercial production, primarily through crossbreeding programmes, as well as to identify and propagate better females for the preservation of precious genetic material. Therefore, crossbreeding will be futile unless superior purebred individuals are used.

Out breeding

Mating individuals those are less closely related to the average of the population. There should be no common ancestor in the lineage of the boar and the females for at least four generations. It is a useful mating strategy for purebred animals. Out breeding, or breeding of unrelated animals, is classified into two types: crossbreeding and grading up. Using out breeding strategy, which includes crossbreeding, selective breeding, and grading up according to necessity, resulting in improved crossbred/graded production performance as well as improved growth rate, reproduction, and production.

Cross breeding

Crossbreeding occurs when two animals of different breeds mate. Mating individuals from different breeds, resulting in a gene combination that is distinct from that found in either parent or in the breed of either parent. Depending on the desired outcome, cross breeding can involve two or more breeds. The main goal of cross breeding is to capitalise on the observed improvement in progeny performance over either parent (hybrid vigour or heterosis).

Effect of Cross Breeding

- A farmer takes a female piglet from a local sow and a male piglet from an exotic sow to his farm for breeding purposes.
- Piglets with larger body sizes are born from the local sow.

- All male piglets are sold, and only a few crossbred females are maintained for breeding.
- Another exotic male unrelated to the herd was introduced for breeding.
- Piglets are born who are very healthy, strong, energetic, and growing quickly.

Criss crossing- It is the alternate use of boars of two breeds on the female stock produced in a herd.

Rotational cross systems combine two or more breeds, where the breed of boar used is different from the previous generation and replacement crossbred females are retained from each cross.

Grading up

Grading up is the breeding of animals of two distinct breeds in which animals of a native breed/genetic group are mated with animals of an improved pure breed for several generations in order to achieve the superior qualities of the improved breed.

Grading up refers to the continuous use of purebred sires of the same breed in a grade herd. By the fifth generation, the graded animals could be close to purebred.

Inbreeding

Mating among members of the same breed who are more closely related than the population average. This could be between full siblings or sire-daughter, mother-son relationships. Pure breeding is a type of in-breeding. Inbreeding has the effect of increasing the proportion of common genes in the progeny. This high prevalence of homozygous gene pairs is true for both desirable and negative features. Several harmful traits, such as hernia and cryptorchidism, include recessive alleles, and inbreeding maintains their phenotypic expression. Inbreeding reduces litter size and raises mortality rates. Inbred sows have poor milking and mothering abilities. It causes gilts and boars to be sexually mature later. Inbred pigs have lower sexual desire.

Breeding Policy in India

- In conjunction with ICAR-NRC on Pig and ICAR-NBAGR, Karnal, all states should take critical measures towards breed registration of indigenous germplasm.
- In its breeding tract, a nucleus breeding farm for such indigenous registered germplasm is required.

- Prized animals may be taken from farmers' fields/state/central government farms and sent to the nucleus herd.
- Animals with pedigrees should be propagated.
- Valuable indigenous animals should not be allowed to crossbreed.
- Those farmers may be eligible for a state department incentive.
- If available, indigenous animals with larger litter sizes and body weights may be employed to improve nondescript animals with appropriate planning.

Breeding with Exotic Germplasm

- Exotic germplasm, particularly Hampshire, Large White Yorkshire, Duroc, Landrace, and Large Black, is imported from a reputable source. The first three breeds for import may be given priority.
- Because frozen semen has a very low success rate, live animals may be imported instead of frozen semen.
- Imported germplasm is used to create a breed-specific nucleus herd for use in a crossbreeding programme.

Crossbred to be propagated in different region

1	Northern India	1.Large White Yorkshire 2.Large White Yorkshire cross 3. Landrace cross
2	Northeastern India	1.Hampshire cross 2.Large white Yorkshire specifically for Mizoram and Tripura 3.Triple cross with Duroc as terminal sire 4.Large Black cross
3	Eastern India	1.Hampshire cross 2.Tamworth cross (specifically Jharkhand)
4	Central India	1. Landrace cross 2. Large White Yorkshire cross
5	Southern India	1. Large White Yorkshire cross 2. Triple cross with Duroc as terminal sire
6	Western India	1. Large White Yorkshire cross

10

Selection of Breeding Stock

The selection of individual animals from a group is very important in a livestock farming business. While creating a herd, every farmer should buy animals from a trustworthy disease-free herd and learn as much as they can about the animals. Once the herd is established, the selection of gilts and boars for replacement in the breeding herd should be based on type and performance. The following are important criteria to consider while creating a healthy sow herd:

- Size of litters
- Strength and vigour of litters
- Milking ability
- Temperament

Economic Traits

Many important production qualities in animals, including body weight, total fat, carcass weight in animals, dressing percentage, and fat content of meat, are quantitative traits, and animal geneticists accomplished most of the research into the patterns of inheritance of these traits. These characteristics are governed by several genes, which segregate according to Mendel's rules. The environment can also influence these features to differing degrees. The following are some examples of economic or quantitative qualities with which we are interested in swine production.

- Litter size at birth
- Litter size born alive
- Litter size at weaning
- Birth weight
- Litter weight at birth
- Litter weight at weaning

- Weight at market age
- Growth rate
- Feed efficiency
- Mortality percentage

Selection of gilts

- Choose breeding gilts at weaning; advanced selection should take place at 5-6 months of age.
- Select weaners that grow quickly. They will almost certainly necessitate less feed per unit live weight gain. As a result, it is less expensive to maintain.
- The breeding herd's final selection of gilts should be made at market weight.
- Choose gilts from sows who have frequently farrowed and weaned large litters.
- They achieved market weight in the shortest amount of time and have a market type.
- It would be preferable to select gilts whose littermates and other fullsibs have demonstrated greater performance in terms of daily weight gain and feed conversion efficiency.
- Gilts should have at least 12-14 teats in order to nurse a large litter.
- Gilts should be selected from sows that wean 9 -10 or more piglets every litter, are good mothers, have their first farrowing at one year of age, and have a seven-month farrowing interval.
- At the time of the first service, the gilt should be at least 8 months old.
- Select gilts with well-developed hams and a tiny head.
- The chosen gilts should have good physical stature, such as strong legs and sound feet.
- Gilt with inverted teats and fat deposited at the base of the teats should not be used for breeding.

Selection of boars

- It is critical to choose a good boar because it gives half of the herd's quality.
- Boar selection is critical, especially for a small breeding farm or unit.
- The boar should be obtained from a breeder or farm that keeps detailed records on its performance.

- The boar should come from a dam that has consistently farrowed and weaned large litters.
- In roughly 5-6 months, a good boar will weigh 90 kg.
- Boars of good type will be sturdy on their feet and legs.

Points to be considered while replacing boars and gilts

- The mother of the pig to be chosen should have had large litters of at least eight weaned piglets.
- In the case of a gilt selection, the weaning weight (at 56 days) of a litter should have been 120 kg, and in the case of a sow, it should not have been less than 150 kg.
- After about 6 months, the gilt or boar should have acquired a body weight of roughly 90 kg.
- The pig's body length and depth should be appropriate, and thick, well-muscled hams should be solid and neat.
- The pig's feet and legs should be sturdy.
- Gilts should have at least 12 teats that are evenly placed and functioning. An animal with blind teats should be avoided since the teats will produce little or no milk and the defect is heritable.
- During selection, animals should be free of brucellosis and leptospirosis, and pigs should be immunised against swine fever.
- Further illnesses and physical deformities in pigs should be avoided.

Breeding methods

- Pen mating, hand mating and artificial insemination are the three important methods of breeding in pig farming. Pen mating is more common on smaller farms.
- Pen mating with a group of newly weaned sows is less common because their estrous cycles may occur close together, resulting in over-use of the boar.
- Hand mating normally involves the female being mated two or three times during estrus, with the first service occurring on the first day of standing estrus and subsequent matings occurring at 24-hour intervals.
- Many farmers would breed the sow or gilt once a day for as long as she accepts the boar. The usage of two separate boars may result in more piglets each litter.

- Heat detection is conducted twice or once per day in AI applications.
- If heat detection is done twice a day, gilts should be inseminated twice, 8-12 hours after the start of standing heat and again 12-16 hours later. Sows should be inseminated 24 hours after standing heat begins and again 18-24 hours later.
- If heat detection is done once per day, gilts should be inseminated within 4 hours and sows should be inseminated within 12-16 hours of being first seen in standing heat. For animals that remain in standing heat, a second insemination should be conducted.
- Single-sire or pooled boar ejaculates extended semen can be used for insemination.
- When specific genetic off spring are required, single-sire matings are under taken, where as pooled semen matings are used to create market hog off spring.

11

Housing Management for Pig

The house should provide adequate protection from direct sunlight and rain. Pigs are extremely sensitive to heat and cold. In rural locations, simple low-cost dwellings built with locally accessible materials are preferred. It is also possible to construct adaptable pens that may be used for all types of pigs. Adequate pig housing is critical for disease prevention, parasite control, and labour savings.

The vital points about the pig house are as follows:

- Build the shed on a dry and adequately raised site.
- Avoid locations that are flooded, swampy, or have a lot of rain.
- The shed's side walls should be 4-5 feet tall, with the remaining height supported by GI pipes or wooden poles.
- Plastering the walls will make them damp proof.
- The roof should be 8-10 feet height.
- The pig stys must be properly aired.
- To stay dry and clean, the floor should be cemented, non-slippery, well sloped, and thoroughly drained.
- Feed troughs, drains, and walls should have rounded corners for easy cleaning.
- Provide plenty of space for each animal.
- In the summer, provide adequate shade and cool drinking water.
- Correctly dispose of faeces and urines.
- Separate pens should be given for boars and lactating sows.
- Group pens can be utilised to house dry sows and fatteners.
- To ensure thermal comfort, provide shade, a wallowing tank, and cooling equipment such as sprinkling water.
- Boars, pregnant, dry sows, gilts, and growing pigs are often housed in open yards with some shade.

- Farrowing sows are housed in completely enclosed pens or homes.
- In huge high-tech farms, individual or group housing in cages built of vertical G.I. pipes, as well as farrowing crates, can be used.
- Males and females who have not been castrated should not be housed together beyond the age of four months.
- The house's floor must be raised around 60 cm above the ground.
- The roof must be waterproof.
- The high side of the roof should face in such a way that some sunlight can enter the home from this side, but there should always be shade in some part of the house.

Selection of housing locations

- The farm should be placed near a city with a high demand for hog products. This is mostly necessary to prevent the costs of transporting feed and other items, as well as the disposal of animals.
- The location should be on a high point that will not be swamped by rainwater.
- The place should be shaded by trees and have plenty of fresh air.
- Away from the residential area.
- In the case of a large pig farm, the site chosen must be adequately connected to roads.
- The site should be suitable for manure disposal and have access to reliable water and electricity.
- Farms should not be established in city areas where health officials may object in the future.
- The structure should be sited so that doors and windows receive maximum sunlight.

Systems of Housing Pigs

Pigs are kept under two systems: (a) Open air system, and (b) Indoor system.

Most farms, though, use a combination of the two. Both of these methods have benefits and drawbacks. The size of the firm, the type of pigs to be produced, and the climatic circumstances all have a role in determining the housing scheme.

Housing and pens for pigs

Pigs in pig sty can be maintained alone or in small groups. When constructing a sty, choose a location that will not flood during the rainy season. The floor should be concrete and slanted away from the sleeping area, allowing urine to flow out and away. The concrete floor should be between 5 and 6 centimetres thick. If the concrete is thin and cracked, the pigs will dig it up quickly. A clay floor cannot be kept clean and will cause parasite and disease concerns. The sty's walls should be smooth so that they can be maintained clean. Dirt and germs can accumulate in cracks in the walls. In the shelter, the animals should have plenty of bedding.

Housing for piglets

Pigs are quite sensitive to temperature extremes. Pigs lack effective heat management mechanisms, and sweating occurs only through the snout. As a result, keeping them cool in hot weather is difficult. Temperature in a pig house is one of the most important elements to consider. Sufficient bedding should be provided to keep the young animals warm, and it should be changed on a regular basis. If a litter is housed in a sty, the sty should be thoroughly cleaned once the litter has been weaned and relocated. If a litter is kept in the field, the shelter should be relocated to a new location for the next litter to avoid disease concerns, especially parasitic worms. Whatever housing arrangement was utilised, piglets should have had access to a warm location that the sow could not reach. There is a crawl area where piglets can be fed and lie down without fear of the mother falling on top of them. By erecting a temporary wall or strong rails, the sow is barred from entering the crawl. This region is typically 0.75 m × 2.4 m in size. The base rail is approximately 30 cm off the ground, allowing the small piglets to travel beneath it. The creep space flooring should have a rough finish and be of a normal sandstone type composed of waterproof cement mortar. Appropriate drains should be installed to dispose of the effluents.

Housing of Boars

Boar pen should have covered area of 6.25-7.5 m^2 and open area of 8.8-12 m^2 for exercise. The walls should have a minimum height of 1.5 m.

Housing of sows

Open yard type with part roofing as in the case of boar may be provided. A total of 10-15 females can be grouped in a pen. An area of 2 m^2 per animal should be provided.

Housing of Farrowing sows

Farrowing sows may be housed independently in a farrowing pen of 2.5 x 4 = 10 m^2 having guard rails, creep area, feed and water troughs.

Housing of growing and finishing pigs

For fatteners, a roofed solid yard for feeding and resting, with a feed and water channel in the front and an open yard will sufficient. The total space necessity may be 2 m^2 per grower/fattener pig.

Wallows

Pigs have a limited number of sweat glands. In places with a warm temperature, mature breeding and fattening animals require a wallow throughout the summer months. It would be ideal to have a brickwork wallow with good drainage. The size of the wallow will be determined by the quantity and size of the animals.

Pigsty

- A pigsty can be built cheaply by utilising locally accessible materials. It must be built in accordance with climatic conditions and the pig production system.
- The pigs should be at ease in their pigsty.
- There is adequate ventilation and shade, no overheating, no odours, and no moisture.
- The structure should be built in an east-west direction.
- The costs of building the pigsty should correspond to the pig production techniques.

The typical floor size, water, and air space requirements in pens for various classes of pigs are listed below.

Class of animals	Covered floor area per animal (m^2)	Open-yard area per animal (m^2)	Water required (litres)	Maximum number of animals per pen
Boar	6.25-7.5	8.8-12.0	15-20	Individual pens
Farrowing pen	7.5-9.0	8.8-12	18-22	Individual pens
Weaner	0.96-1.8	8.8-12	3.5-4	30
Dry sow/gilt	1.8-2.7	1.4-1.8	4.5-5	3-10
Fattener (3-5 months old)	0.9-1.2	0.9-1.2	10-12	30
Fattener (above five months)	1.3-1.8	1.3.1.8	12-15	30

12

Digestive System of The Pig

The digestive mechanism of a pig is ideally adapted to full concentrate-based meals. The digestive organs are quite simple, with a continuous musculo-membanous tube from the mouth to the anus. However, this system includes multiple sophisticated interaction functions.

Mouth

The mouth is necessary not only for food consumption, but also for first partial size reduction by grinding. While teeth are the major means of reducing meal size and increasing surface area, when feed is mixed with saliva, the first step in the chemical breakdown of food occurs. The three primary salivary glands are the parotid, mandibular, and sublingual glands. Saliva secretion is a reflex activity that occurs when there is food in the mouth. The amount of mucus in saliva is determined by the wetness or dryness of the meal consumed. As a result, on a dry diet, more saliva mucus is secreted, whereas on a moist diet, only enough is secreted to aid in swallowing. Amylase, the enzyme that hydrolyzes starch to maltose, is present in saliva in very low amounts. Salivary digestive enzymes provide a minor effect. Food is chewed and mixed with saliva before going to the stomach via the mouth, throat, and oesophagus. Oesophageal movement involves muscle peristalsis, or the contraction and relaxation of muscles to move food.

Stomach

The stomach is a muscular organ that stores food, breaks it down, and transfers it to the small intestine. The stomach is separated into four distinct sections: oesophageal, cardiac, fundic, and pyloric. The oesophageal area is located at the confluence of the stomach and the oesophagus. This region of the stomach does not produce digestive enzymes, yet it is important since it is where ulcers develop in pigs. Irritation in this area induced by fine particle size, stress, or other environmental factors can all lead to the production of swine ulcers. After passing through this region, food enters the cardiac zone.

In the cardiac portion of the stomach, mucus is released and mixed with digested food. Food then reaches the fundic region, the first major portion of the stomach where digestion takes place. In this region, gastric glands secrete hydrochloric acid, resulting in a pH of 1.5 to 2.5. The lower pH kills bacteria that are swallowed with the diet. Digestive enzymes, notably pepsinogen, are also secreted in this location. Pepsinogen is then destroyed by hydrochloric acid to produce pepsin, a protein degrading enzyme.

The digesta eventually reaches the pyloric region at the bottom of the stomach. This region is responsible for secreting mucus to line the digestive membranes and protect them from damage caused by the low pH digesta as it travels through the small intestine. The phloric sphincter regulates the amount of digesta that enters the small intestine. This is an important function because it prevents digesta excess in the small intestine, which allows for better digestion and nutrient absorption. Additionally, after leaving the stomach, the digesta is highly fluid.

Small Intestine, Pancreas and Liver

The principal area of nutrition absorption is the small intestine, which is divided into three sections. The first part is the duodenum. The duodenum is a 12-inch-long portion of the small intestine that houses pancreatic and liver ducts. The pancreas is in charge of exocrine and endocrine excretions. The pancreas is in charge of secreting insulin and glucagon in response to high or low blood glucose levels. Exocrine actions include the secretion of digesting enzymes and sodium bicarbonate.

Digestive enzymes secreted into the chyme hydrolyze proteins, lipids, and carbohydrates. Additionally, sodium bicarbonate is required to provide alkalinity so that chyme can be transported into the small intestine without causing cell damage as a result of the low pH after departing the stomach. The pancreas is the most important organ in the digestive process, producing and secreting enzymes essential for chyme digestion and protecting cells from pH damage.

In addition to pancreatic secretions, bile, which is stored in the gall bladder and produced by the liver, is emptied into the duodenum. Bile salts, the active component of bile in the digestive process, aid in fat digestion and absorption but also in the absorption of fat-soluble vitamins and pancreatic lipase in the small intestine. Finally, bile salts are necessary for cholesterol absorption in the lower small intestine.

Once the chyme travels through the duodenum, digestion occurs. The jejunum enters the small intestine's core segment after leaving the duodenum. This region of the small intestine is in charge of subsequent nutritional breakdown as well as the commencement of nutrient absorption. Nutritional absorption continues into the ileum, the small intestine's last section. In the jejunum and ileum, nutrients are absorbed through the brush border, also known as the intestinal mucosa. The mucosa is composed of finger-like projections known as villi, which are composed of smaller projections known as microvilli. The microvilli tips form web-like structures known as glycocalyx.

Amino acids and simple carbohydrates released into the brush border membrane are absorbed by the microvilli first, then the villi, and lastly the circulatory system. Absorbed amino acids and simple carbohydrates are transported straight to the liver via the portal vein. Dietary fat that is broken down and absorbed into the brush border enters the lymphatic system before exiting the lymphatic system and entering the general circulation via the thoracic duct.

Large Intestine

The large intestine, also referred to as the hindgut, is divided into four sections. The digesta from the small intestine enters the caecum first. The caecum is separated into two sections, with the first having a blind end through which no material can flow. A second caecum segment connects to the colon, where digesta is transmitted to the rectum and anus, where the remaining digesta is evacuated.

The fundamental function of the large intestine is water absorption. The chyme that travels from the small intestine and into the large intestine is initially quite fluid. The large intestine epithelium has a high capacity for water absorption.

As digesta moves from the ileum and into the large intestine, there is no enzymatic digestion. However, the large intestine has limited microbial enzyme activity, which results in the creation of VFAs (volatile fatty acids). They are quickly absorbed in the big intestine. In general, they provide only enough energy to meet the dietary needs of the large intestine epithelium. Furthermore, B-vitamins are synthesised in the large intestine and absorbed in very little amounts, insufficient to alter nutritional intake.

After the majority of the water has been eliminated, the digesta condenses into a semi-solid mass and flows out of the rectum and anus.

13

Pig Nutrition

Proper feed is necessary for development, body maintenance, and the production of meat and milk. When correctly prepared, one can use less expensive locally available feeds that are nutritionally sufficient. Pigs can be fed effectively with leftovers from a family's kitchen. Pig nutritional needs can be divided into six sections. Examples include water, carbohydrates, fats, proteins, vitamins, and minerals.

Pigs are omnivorous, which means they can consume both meat and plants. Pigs' digestive systems can also manage roughage-rich diets. Pig must drink plenty of clean, fresh water every day. Pigs will consume practically anything. They will consume grass and other plants. They can be kept in a safe field where they will consume all vegetation and grass. The pig will burrow into the ground and consume both the roots and the green parts of plants. A pig with a nose ring cannot root plants. Pigs will develop and fatten more quickly if fed concentrate feed. Grain meal that has been thoroughly pulverised is a good feed for pig.

Pigs can also be fed leftover veggies and scraps from the kitchen. Before feeding scraps to the pig, household scraps, especially those containing meat, must be well prepared. The pig requires constant access to fresh, clean water. Each day, a sow with young requires 20 to 30 litres of water.

How often will a pig need feeding?

Pigs can be kept in stalls if they are fed twice a day, once in the morning and once in the evening. Pigs in the field can be fed once a day or given extra feed, such as vegetable waste or swill, if it is available. Piglets exhibit an interest in solid food when they are 1 or 2 weeks old. To begin, a handful of cereal, sugar, or powdered milk might be given to them. Piglets will consume mother's milk until they are approximately 7 weeks old. They will gradually consume less milk and more solid nutrition until they are weaned. Piglets in the field will eat solid feed on their own, but those in captivity must be provided it. To avoid gastrointestinal problems, the young animals must be gradually exposed to a new food. A pig's meal should be consumed rapidly. A lack of interest in feed indicates disease, and you must check the animal to determine the cause.

What one shouldn't feed to your pig: Any raw and uncooked carcass or part of a carcass of mammal or bird. This includes any meat blood, offal, hide or feathers. Pigs that feed on carcasses are also at risk of contracting diseases that are infectious to humans.

Feeding management

- Pigs are monogastric animals that can only consume a limited amount of fibrous food. Mature pigs digest fibrous food more efficiently than young stock.
- A portion of the protein in pigs' diets should come from animal sources.
- Pigs should be fed on frequent basis.
- New feed should be added only after the old feed has been finished or removed.
- In the case of swill feeding, the pig requires 4-8 kg of swill per day on average.
- Pigs can be given a modest amount of feed.
- To avoid post-weaning weight depression, weaned pigs can be fed ad libitum using an automatic feeder.
- Provide enough concentrates in the ration.
- Give enough vitamins and minerals.
- Make sure there is enough clean water.
- The feeding of the piglets is more crucial, and high-quality, enriched diets are required.
- Feeding sows during pregnancy is critical for raising litter size.
- The feed requirements of a lactating sow should be determined by the litter size, weight, size, and age of the sow.
- To lower production costs, commercial pig farming should prepare for the use of nontraditional feed supplies, such as waste from kitchens/hotels/ cold storage, in place of balanced diets.
- The feeding system chosen should meet all of the nutrient requirements of the various pig types.
- Any abrupt changes in animal feed can result in a loss of productivity. As a result, feed modifications should be made as gradually as feasible.

- To prevent overturning and waste of feed, the feeding dish should be securely fastened to the floor.
- Water can also be provided by the feeding trough. Automatic drinkers are utilised on large farms.

Types of Pig Feed

To offer the best nutrition possible for pigs, feeds must be tailored to their specific requirements at various ages and phases of production. Pig feed comes in six varieties. They are:

1. Creep Feed
2. Weaner Feed
3. Grower Feed
4. Fattener Feed
5. Pregnant Sow Feed
6. Lactating Sow Feed

1. **Creep Feed:** Creep feeding is the process of self-feeding concentrates to young piglets in a separate environment apart from their mother. This is a specific type of feed that is given to suckling piglets aged 2 to 8 weeks. Piglets can be fed creep feed 7 to 10 days after birth.
2. **Weaner Feed:** This pig food is designed specifically for young, weaned piglets weighing 6 weeks to 20 kg.
3. **Grower Feed:** This food is intended for young pigs weighing more than 20 kg or aged 10 weeks until they reach a body weight of 35 to 40 kg. This feed must be given before the fattener feed is supplied.
4. **Fattener Feed:** This feed is given to pigs weighing more than 40 kg until they reach a marketable body weight of 90-100 kg.
5. **Pregnant Sow Feed:** This feed is intended for pregnant sows and can be fed to boars weighing more than 90 kg.
6. **Lactating Sow Feed:** This meal is designed specifically for lactating sows.

The best technique to feed farm animals is to make the whole diet prescribed for each class and give the pigs the quantity they will eat without waste two or three times per day. The pigs will consume around the following amount of dry feed.

Age (wks)	Body Weight (kg)	Feed kg/day
8-10	12-15	0.66
10-12	15-20	0.1
12-16	20-40	2.0
16-18	40-50	2.5
18-24	50-84	3.0
24-28	84-105	3.5

Ground grains should be used in all mixed feeds. Wet mash feeding is not usually superior to slop/dry feeding. Slop feeding necessitates more time and effort. Pelletizing feed may boost the rate and effectiveness of weight growth if the ration is high in fibre. Pelleting may help reduce the amount of lost feed.

It is critical not to overfeed sows that have been bred. Overweight sows are more likely to produce frail pigs and crush more piglets during farrowing. From breeding until farrowing, sows should acquire about 35 kg and gilts should gain about 55 kg.

Miscellaneous feeds which can be fed to pigs: Swill (kitchen waste, including leftover human food, vegetables, meat, and fish cuts) Check to ensure that the swill feed is not too old and putrefied. Each pig requires 4 to 8 kg of swill per day on average.

Other feeds used for feeding pig

Item	Incorporation level up to (%)
Tapioca starch waste	15-20
Rubber seed cake	15
Tamarind seed roasted	20
Meat offal	20

Feeding of growing and finishing pigs

Pigs may be given comprehensive diet to promote optimal growth. They could be fed at least twice or three times every day. The typical post-weaning feed conversion efficiency till market weight is roughly 4, suggesting that the pig would consume this much feed to gain one kilogramme of weight. It varies widely, though, depending on age and ambient temperature. Protein needs are greater during early stage. When fattening progresses, the protein content in the diet may decrease.

Boar, sow, and castrates can all be fattened for meat. Growers should be classified as uniformly as possible based on sex, size, and weight. The weight difference between small and large pigs in a lot should not exceed 20%.

A pig pen may easily house up to 15 pigs. Sprinklers, wallowing tanks, and other cooling equipment, in addition to shade, may be provided in the heat. Poorly performing growers should be identified, culled, and removed from the lot as soon as feasible. Deworming can be done two weeks after weaning and should be done every two months if necessary.

Feeding of boars

A breeding pig requires 2-2.5 kilogramme concentrate per 100 kg weight, depending on age, condition, and breeding drive. Feed allowances should be controlled to prevent the pig from becoming obese or exhausted. Greens should be provided if kept indoors. Year-round pasture is excellent if it can be provided to provide both exercise and nutrients.

Feeding of female

Feeding should be carefully monitored to ensure that sows and gilts are never overweight or underweight. Personalised feeding is advised. Flushing is a procedure that involves boosting the diets of sows and gilts for 1-2 weeks prior to mating and then reverting to normal nutrition after mating. The rigours of pregnancy and the need to store calories for eventual nursing are accelerated during the final stages of pregnancy.

Feeding of Farrowing Sow and Litter

Feed cautiously before and after farrowing with bulky laxative feed. The swine will be completely fed after 10 days. Estimated feed allotment is 2.5-3 kg/100 kg body weight plus 0.2 kilogramme feed per piglet produced by the sow. A sow weighing 100 kg with 8 piglets need 4.6 kg of feed each day. The piglets can be fed a special nutritional diet known as creep feed separately.

Orphan pigs

When a sow dies, fails to supply milk, or fails to claim her piglets, the piglets should be shifted as quickly as possible to a foster mother. Some sows may be unwilling to nurse piglets from different sows. When bringing piglets to a foster mother or another suckling sow, it is important to mimic the conditions, including odour and body size. If a suckling sow is not available, hand feeding is essential. Cow's milk is the finest substitute for sow's milk. Buttermilk or sweet skim milk can also be used. Every piglet can have 300-500 mL of milk every day. Feed 5-6 times a day for the first few weeks for the optimum outcomes, then gradually reduce to 2-3 times. Piglings can be given any ordinary vitamin preparation, until they start eating. Injectable iron preparations (such as Imferon) can be used normally.

Pigs can be fed a variety of feed formulae, and the type of feed that is most suited to a specific pig will vary depending on the pig's age, weight, and developmental stage. Most pig farmers will use a range of different diets to ensure that their pigs get all of the nutrients they need.

Pig Starter or Creep Feed Formula

Ingredient	Quantity (kg)
Maize	550
Groundnut Cake (GNC)	140
Brewers Dry Grains (BDG)	133
Soybean Meal (SBM)	90
Fish meal	50
Bone meal	31
Salt	2.5
Methionine	1
Pig Premix	2.5
Total	1000

Pig Grower Feed Formula

Ingredient	Quantity (kg)
Maize	250
Groundnut Cake (GNC)	80
Cassava peels	100
Brewers Dry Grains (BDG)	150
Wheat Offal	274
Soybean Meal (SBM)	50
Palm Kernel Cake (PKC)	62
Bone meal	28
Salt	2.5
Methionine	1
Pig Premix	2.5
Total	1000

Pig Fattener Feed Formula

Ingredient	Quantity (kg)
Maize	220
Groundnut Cake (GNC)	30
Cassava peels	100

Brewers Dry Grains (BDG)	130
Wheat Offal	274
Maize Bran	50
Soybean Meal (SBM)	20
Palm Kernel Cake (PKC)	150
Bone meal	20
Salt	2.5
Methionine	1
Pig Premix	2.5
Total	1000

Pig Breeder Feed Formula

Ingredient	**Quantity (kg)**
Maize	200
Groundnut Cake (GNC)	30
Cassava peels	100
Brewers Dry Grains (BDG)	150
Wheat Offal	299
Maize bran	15
Soybean Meal (SBM)	50
Palm Kernel Cake (PKC)	120
Bone meal	30
Salt	2.5
Methionine	1
Pig Premix	2.5
Total	1000

The composition of the concentrate feed for various age groups pigs

Ingredients	**Creep feed (14th to 56th da**	**Grower ration (up to 40 kg)**	**Finisher ration (40-90 kg)**	**Pregnant and nursing sows**
Maize or sorghum or broken wheat, broken rice and barley in convenient combinations	65	50	50	50

Oil cakes (groundnut oil cake, soya bean oil-cake, sesame oil cake, linseed oil cake	14	18	20	20
Molasses	5	5	5	5
Wheat bran or rice bran	10	1.5	25	18
Fishmeal or meat meal or cooked offal, skim milk powder dairy wastes	5	5	3	5
Mineral mixture	1	1.5	1.5	1
Salt	-	0.5	0.5	0.5

Points to be considered while formulating feeding ration

- The most cost-effective ingredients should be chosen.
- Grains such as maize, sorghum, oats, various millets, wheat, and rice should be the primary constituents.
- Protein supplements include oil cakes, fishmeal, and beef meal.
- If the pigs are permitted to pasture or are given fresh green legumes, vitamin supplements are not required. If no or little animal protein is given, a vitamin B12 supplement might be required.
- Mineral supplements should be available.

Traditional Feed Processing

To make pig feed more appealing; various feeds are blended and boiled. Combining all of the different feeds together in proportion (rice bran, broken rice, crushed maize and soya, dried legume leaves, etc.) and feeding it directly to the pigs.

Different feed ingradients for pig ration formulation

Rice Bran: This is excellent for pig feeding. It has 11% protein content and can be utilised as the main ingredient in most meals. Rice bran can be combined with other feeds in amounts ranging from 30 to 45%. However, it should not be kept for longer than a month because it will mould.

Maize: This is an excellent animal feed. It can hold up to 65% carbs and 9% protein. It can be combined with other feeds, but not more than 40% of the total ration.

Wheat Bran: This is high in dietary fibre and contains significant amounts of carbohydrate, protein, vitamins, and minerals. Wheat Bran is widely utilised as a primary ingredient in animal feed. It contains 14% - 16% protein, 9.5% fat, 8 - 10% crude fibre, and up to 25% carbohydrate.

Root Crops: This can be blended with other feeds in amounts ranging from 10% to 30%, but never more than 30%. Before using, the crop should be peeled and washed, then sliced, dried, and ground. The dried cassava can be stored for a longer period of time. Because of the toxic chemicals present, raw cassava with the skin should not be fed to pigs.

Vegetables: Vegetables that have been damaged during shipment, storage, and handling can be used as a supplement feed for pigs by boiling them and mixing them with other feeds such rice bran, broken rice, and maize. Cauliflower, lettuce, spinach, morning glory, sweet potato vine, cola-cassia (requires boiling), pumpkin, guords, and water hyacinth are all appropriate veggies.

Cola-cassia/Pandalu: Pigs may obtain protein from the leaves and stems. Leaves include 20% of the dietary dry matter and 46% of the crude protein after heating. It also contains a lot of calcium, phosphorus, iron, Vitamin C, thiamine, riboflavin, and niacin, which are all important nutrients for pigs. The fresh tuber contains about 20% dry matter, whereas the fresh petiole contains just about 6% dry matter. Because of their high crude protein content, the leaves and stems are employed as a local protein source for pig production.

Banana Stem: Because fresh green banana or plantain fruits are low in organic nutrients, chopping them and sprinkling salt on the slices is the best way to feed them. This is a favourite of pigs. Green bananas or plantains are preferred for ensiling over ripe fruits, which lose some of their dry matter and, more importantly, sugars during the process.

Alfalfa: Despite its low fibre level, alfalfa is appealing to pigs and easy to digest. It is the most complete nutritional combination one can feed to pigs. It also has 47 vital elements and one of nature's most generous vitamin, mineral, and amino acid balances.

Mulberry: The protein and dry matter content of fresh mulberry leaf foliage is well utilised by growing pigs fed a base diet of broken rice.

Forest products can also be used to make pig feed. Food waste can also be utilised. The following ingredients are typically combined with distillery waste: rice bran/wheat bran (2 kg), broken rice (1 kg), distillers' residues

(5-10 kg), and other locally accessible agricultural by-products. Alcohol can be made from millet, rice, maize, sweet potato, yam, banana, and other native grains. The most widely used distillery waste for pig feeding is millet and rice waste; the protein content ranged from 17 to 33% on a dry matter basis. It should be mixed with other feed items such as rice bran, wheat bran, maize/millet flour, and broken rice. Distillery wastes can be fed to fattening pigs but not pregnant or nursing sows. These animals, however, require high quality diet; hence distillery waste must be supplemented with other high quality feed, such as commercial feeds.

All pigs require enough clean drinking water.

A pregnant sow requires 10 - 12 litres of water per day.

A lactating sow requires 20 – 30 litres of water per day.

A growing pig requires 6 - 8 liters of water per day.

A boar requires 12 - 15 liters of water per day.

Pigs' daily feed intake will be reduced if they are not given enough water. Pigs must have access to sufficient clean water at all times.

14

Pig Farm Management

Pig Identification

Animal identification is very important aspect on any livestock farm. Some types of identity are merely temporary, dissipating after a few days. Temporary identification, such as a grease paint stick, can be used to identify certain pigs within a pen, such as when immunisation pigs.

Some forms of identification are more durable. Ear tags are commonly used. Some producers use plastic tags with numbers to help them identify individual pigs. Pigs, on the other hand, are inquisitive creatures who frequently consider a plastic tag on another pig as an intriguing toy. Plastic tags are commonly torn and misplaced as a result. Additionally, when the tag punctures the ear, pigs frequently develop an ear infection. Tiny metal tags may be used, but they are subject to the same long-term loss and infection problems.

The most lasting method of identification used by most manufacturers is ear notching. In this procedure, little notches are carved into the baby pigs' ears right after birth using a small pair of v-shaped pliers. The notches represent numbers and will accompany the pig for the remainder of its life. Farmers may develop their own ear-notching system, but the universal ear notching system is the most widely used.

Pig record keeping

There are five reasons for producing information:

1. To improve overall efficiency.
2. To increase profitability.
3. To know performance level of your farm
   - Production levels.
   - Reproduction levels.

- Management achievements.
- Economics.
- The use of feeds.
- Growth performance.
- The levels of disease.
- The levels of medicinal treatment.

4. For epidemiological studies.
5. Aids for daily management.

Management decisions are influenced by three major factors: economics, production, and feed. The overall liveweight of pigs leaving the farm determines profitability. Every kilogramme of liveweight sold increases the profit margin over feed while incurring just little additional costs. Another crucial management decision is matching the right pig to the right market.

Each sow, sucking pig, weaner, and grower-finisher data are utilised to monitor productivity, as are disease, treatment, and death levels for each of these animals.

Feed utilisation is the third recording area and the most expensive, therefore tracking expenses per tonne, liveweight gain prices, and efficiency of use is vital. It is here that records and computer technology can be used most efficiently, yet it is also typically where there is the least input.

What should be recorded

Make a note of this information for each female:

- Tag number
- weaning to oestrus interval
- Date and time of proestrus
- Date, time and duration of oestrus
- Date and time of first standing heat
- Variations in the number of days between weaning and oestrus, and oestrus duration
- Seasonal changes
- Date and time of all inseminations
- Projected and actual return dates
- Weaning to service interval for your breeding herd

- Review recorded information regularly to determine any trends for your farm or for individual females
- Tailor the insemination routine accordingly
- Any other observations

Handling the young pig

By holding the rear leg just above the hock, piglets can be grasped and held from behind. Pulling the piglet needs placing the second hand beneath the animal's chest and lifting it. When holding the piglet, always support its weight against you. By the time the piglet is weaned, it will be too hefty to lift.

Handling the older pig

As one approach or attempt to catch a pig, it will seek a gap. This habit can be used to direct the pig's movements. The pig will move forward in the direction requested by the handlers if two pig boards (0.8m square wooden planks) are placed either side of its head. When the animal grows older, it can be taught to move with the help of a board and a 1 m long wooden bat by a single operator. Always keep the pig board between the handler and the pig.

Restraining a pig

A pig can be restrained by tying it with ropes to a wall or fence. Large pigs can be easily restrained with a rope or wire loop around the snout.

Castrating piglets

Male pigs have the ability to fight and hurt one another. Castrated pigs are quieter and easier to manage. Castrating the pig allows it to gain weight and the meat to lose its distinctive piggy odour. Castration should be performed on young pigs between the ages of 2 and 3 weeks.

Restraining the pig for castration

- During castration, someone must hold the piglet. The pig should be supported by its back legs, with its head down and its torso securely held between the handler's knees.
- It will be necessary to use an exceptionally sharp, clean knife, scalpel, or razor blade. Remove the sow from the litter and, if possible, relocate her to a location where she will not be able to see or hear them. Rinse and dry the scrotum with warm water and soap.
- Put your finger into the scrotum, then use your thumb and index finger to firmly grip the scrotum underneath the testicle.

- In the scrotum, make a 1 to 2 cm long incision. The testicle should come out of the wound.
- Cut through the white cord, leaving the red blood artery intact, then remove the testicle from the scrotum.
- Pull the testicle out further and twist it numerous times before severing the twisted blood vessel with a knife scraped up and down. This assists in reducing bleeding. Do not tug so hard that you damage the vessel.
- Never, ever stick your fingers into your scrotum. Use an iodine tincture, gentian violet, Dettol, antibiotic powder, or sulpha powder on the castration wound. Remove the second testicle in the same way.
- The piglets and their mother should have clean bedding. Keep a watch out for signs of infection in the piglets' wounds during the next week.

Teeth clipping in young pigs

Piglets bite the sow as they compete for one of her teats. The pain disturbs the sow, causing her to stand up and prevent her young from feeding. With the incisions, germs have the ability to penetrate the sow's udder. When they compete for the teat and suckle, piglets will bite and damage one another. These complications can be avoided by just cutting the teeth as soon as possible after birth.

When to clip the teeth

The piglet's teeth should be cut as soon as possible after birth. The sow and her young should be separated for as little a time as feasible. Tooth clippers, pliers, or forceps will be needed to clip the teeth.

Clipping the teeth

- If the sow is not tethered, separate her from her young and place her in another pen. Take precautions because the sow with a litter could be dangerous.
- Gather the young pigs and place them in a box.
- To open the piglet's jaws, hold its head and press the corner of its mouth.
- Place the clippers on either side of one pair of teeth, keeping the tongue clear. Tilt head back and let the tooth fragments fall out of mouth.
- Trim the teeth as close to the gum line as possible.
- Clean the clippers before using them on another piglet. Operate on the rest of the litter before returning the piglets to their mother. Warm the young pigs up.

Removal of needle teeth

Piglets are born with four razor-sharp pairs of teeth, two on each jaw. They offer no practical value to the piglets and may irritate the sow's udder or damage other piglets during nursing. If the needle teeth are trimmed immediately after birth, the udder will be safeguarded.

Anaemia in piglets

Piglet anaemia is a common dietary disorder. Iron can be given orally or intravenously to prevent and treat this condition. Piglets suffer from severe anaemia due to a shortage of iron and copper in sow's milk. Impacted piglets become weak, dyspeptic, and have difficulty breathing. Because of their difficulties breathing, this illness is commonly referred to as thumps. To prevent piglet anaemia, swab a sow's udder with a saturated solution of ferrous sulphate to ensure that piglets obtain these minerals while drinking milk. This solution must be applied everyday from birth until the piglets begin taking creep feed. Injection of commercially available iron-dextran complexes is another effective approach.

Flushing

It is the practise of providing food to sows and gilts before to breeding. A high-quality grower food given to sows and gilts seven to ten days before breeding promotes increased ovulation rates. Following breeding, sows and gilts should be fed a restricted but well-balanced diet until the last six weeks of pregnancy, when full feeding should resume.

Care and management of sow

Sow care and management are crucial because they are primarily kept in the herd for breeding. With correct management and feed, breeding challenges can be reduced. Sows should be given extra care so that the piglets are born normally and nursed properly.

Care during Pregnancy

Sow is pregnant if sow is not in heat three weeks after mating. The pregnancy will last three months, three weeks, and three days. During pregnancy, the sow will require a high-nutrient diet, especially near the end of the pregnancy. She should be fed a nutrient-dense meal every day, such as grains and greenstuffs. When the time comes for the sow to give birth, make sure she has enough of clean bedding.

One week before farrowing, give pregnant sows additional attention by providing adequate space, feed, and water. Three to four days before the expected date of farrowing, disinfect the sows and farrowing pens, and then place the sows in the farrowing pen after properly bedding it.

Sow gestation lasts from 109 and 120 days, with an average of 114 days. To reduce fighting, which can lead to abortion, pregnant animals should be housed in groups in separate cages and not combined with new animals. Pregnant gilts and sows should be housed in separate groups during gestation. Each sow should have a dry housing area of about 3 m^2. Pregnant animals should be allowed to move about on a free range or, if available, a pasture every morning. It is thought that a cultivated crop growing in the pasture is clean.

Farrowing Sow and Litter

Signs that the pig is ready to farrow

The sow becomes restless and begins to build a nest within 24 hours of giving birth. The teat will produce milk when gently squeezed.

Blood-tinged fluid may be produced from the vagina, 1 to 2 hours before birth, and if small greenish pellets appear, the first piglet will arrive within an hour.

Normal farrowing

Farrowing is a natural procedure in which the sow does not usually require help. The others, as well as the afterbirth, will arrive shortly after the first piglet is born. Farrowing should take about 2 to 3 hours. The navel cord will snap, and the piglet will immediately seek a teat and milk. If the navel bleeds, tie it tightly with a clean string or rope.

When and how to help in farrowing

- If the sow shows all indicators of farrowing but has not delivered a piglet and is pawing with a rear leg, or if 45 minutes have passed and no sign of the second piglet has developed, one must assist the sow.
- Warm water and soap should be used to scrub beneath your fingernails and to wash your hands and arms.
- Clean the vulva area.
- Hands should be washed with soap or rubbed with olive or sunflower oil.
- Put your hand inside the vagina and try to remove the tissue or debris that is creating the obstruction.
- Clear the mucus from the piglet's mouth and nostrils, and slap it if it isn't breathing. Dry the piglet gently and place its mouth on a teat.
- Let the farrowing pen to dry for a week after cleaning and disinfecting it with a 2% phenyl lotion solution.

- The pregnant female should be dewormed 2-3 weeks before to farrowing and before being admitted to the farrowing pen. Spray with an external parasiticide (1% malathion/cythion solution, butox. 0.05%). Clean the undersurface, sides, interdigital space, and udder with soap and water soon before moving into the farrowing pen to eliminate filth, parasite eggs, disease germs, and so on.
- Move the clean animal to the clean pen ten days before farrowing.
- Provide mild bedding of chopped straw 2-3 days before farrowing.
- As teats are pressed, milk appears, indicating that farrowing time is near.
- Keep an eye on the farrowing the entire time. It may persist up to 24 hours.
- With a towel or straw, clean the piglets. To disinfect the naval chord, apply iodine tincture. Teats are suckled within 10-30 minutes by normal healthy piglets. Aid small piglets in sucking.
- Placenta, dead piglets, unclean bedding, and other such items should be removed and buried as quickly as possible. The placenta is normally released within a few days.
- To avoid piglet anaemia, administer 50 mg iron (Imferon 1 ml) intramuscularly on the second day. Oral administration of iron solution (1 g Ferrous sulphate in 25 ml of water) 1 ml per piglet once a week can be tried. A second injection may be administered at the age of 5 weeks.
- Maintain a warm, dry, and clean farrowing pen.
- Needle teeth can be carefully extracted.
- The time necessary for litter expulsion ranges between 1 and 5 hours. The interval between the first and subsequent piglets' births spans from a few minutes to three hours. A posterior presentation occurs in approximately 30% of piglets. The placenta is usually released only after all of the piglings have been delivered. Normally, the placenta is released three hours after the foetus is discharged. Suckling begins within the first 10-15 minutes of life. To avert mortality from chilling during the cold and wet seasons, artificial heat can be produced using an infrared lamp or an ordinary electric bulb.

Management at farrowing

Farrowing is an important stage in pig production. The death rate during farrowing and the first week after farrowing is high. Farrowing pens with guard rails and a creep space, as well as farrowing crates or stalls, can be used for sows. It is sufficient to have a pen with guard rails and a crawl space. The temperature in the pen should be kept between 24°C and 28°C until the piglets are three or four days old, and then between 18°C and 22°C until the piglets are six weeks old. Heat lamps should be hung 45 centimetres off the ground and completely covered. The farrowing pens should be well cleaned before bringing in the sow. This will help to prevent a variety of piglet diseases.

The sow should be introduced to the farrowing pen at least one week before farrowing to familiarise herself with the environment. Before being transferred to the farrowing pen, she should be thoroughly cleansed. The feed ration should be bulked up by replacing one-third of the conventional ration with wheat bran. Decrease the ration supply by one-third until the sow farrows. The sow should be watched regularly to establish the approximate time of farrowing, and no feed should be given 12 hours before farrowing.

Care during farrowing

An attendant should be present when the sow farrows. Otherwise, a large number of piglets will perish. On average, farrowing takes between 2 and 4 hours. The piglets should be taken as they farrow and kept warm in the creep chamber until the procedure is finished. Each piglet should be cleaned of any mucus to ensure that the breathing passageways are clear. The navel cord should be tied 2-5 cm away from the navel, severed with sanitised scissors, and the stumps iodine-painted. Piglets should be allowed to nurse after birth. After around 2 days, they settle down to their specific teats. They nurse 8-10 times in 24 hours in the initial period. Trampling by the sow should be prevented during the first two weeks.

Care of Piglets

- The piglets are taken as they farrow and kept warm in the creep space until the farrowing process is completed.
- To ensure that the breathing passage is clear, each piglet is cleaned for all the mucus.
- The navel cord should be tied 2.5 cm away from the navel, and the remainder should be removed hygienically.
- Iodine tincture can be used to treat and disinfect the navel cord.
- Provide guard rails to protect newly born piglets.
- After birth, piglets should be breastfed. They nurse 8 to 10 times per day.
- Give sows' milk together with creep feed for the first 6-8 weeks.
- Safeguard the piglets from harsh weather, especially during the first two months.

- Needle teeth should be trimmed as soon as possible after delivery.
- Vaccinate the piglets according to the prescribed timetable.
- Iron supplementation is required to prevent piglet anaemia.
- Piglets intended for sale as breeding stock must be appropriately reared.
- Male piglets not selected for breeding should be castrated, preferably at the age of 3-4 weeks, to prevent boar odour in cooked flesh, allowing for the production of high-quality meat.
- Increased feed needs of a lactating sow must be met to guarantee effective breastfeeding of all piglets born.

Fostering piglets

Some piglets are born smaller than others and do not grow quickly. They are hungry, and the smaller piglets grow slowly or die. Expect weight gain and growth disparities among litter members, but if all of the piglets do not grow well and there are no evident signs of illness, the mother's milk production will be minimal. This is especially common in elderly sows. Fostering the piglets, which entails placing them with a different sow for food, may be necessary.

Colostrum from their mothers is required for all piglets. Within one hour of birth, they will take their first feed. If a sow dies during the farrowing process, her litter can be fed to another sow. To make the orphans acceptable to the sow, they should be mixed in with her litter. The foster mother, however, will be unable to feed both litters at the same time, necessitating the necessity for additional foster mothers to feed the orphans.

Raising orphan piglets

- Orphan piglets can be raised either with a foster sow or the use of milk replacer.
- Orphan pigs are the result of a sow's mortality after farrowing, mastitis, and lactation failure of litters larger than the sow's capacity to raise. If another sow has recently farrowed, the orphaned piglets could be transferred to her. This transfer must be accomplished within a few days of farrowing since unutilized areas of the sow's udder quickly stop producing milk. To ensure that new pigs are welcomed, the sow should be separated from her own litter for a short time before introducing the new piglets, and a disinfectant or other material should be sprinkled on all the piglets to mask odours.
- Orphan piglets can also be nursed using milk replacer. To manufacture milk replacer, one egg yolk is thoroughly mixed with one litre of cow milk.

With the exception of iron, this combination provides a well-balanced diet. To compensate for the iron deficiency, add one eighth teaspoon of ferrous sulphate to one litre of milk. An iron compound injection could also be used.

Hand rearing piglets

- A piglet may die if no foster mother is available. Hand feeding can be used to rear the litter. The following items will be required to hand rear a litter:
- Bottles and nipples that have been thoroughly cleaned between feedings.
- A clean, dry box with clean bedding for newborn piglets to keep warm.
- Feedings must be provided every 1 to 2 hours.
- Cow's colostrum is the best substitute for sow's colostrum, and after 3 to 4 days, the piglets can be given milk.

Weaning of piglets

Weaning is normally completed after 7-8 weeks. To reduce weaning stress, the sow should be separated from the piglets for a few hours each day and its nutrition gradually reduced. To avoid weaning stress, separate the sow from the piglets for a few hours each day, and gradually reduce nutrition. The piglets should be dewormed two weeks after weaning. The piglets should be gradually moved from an 18% protein creep diet to a 16% grower ration over the course of two weeks. Each pen should house a group of 20 piglets of similar ages.

When to wean piglets

It should be noted that weaning time varies depending on the type of pig breed. Piglets will show social cues indicating when it is time to wean. Watch out for the following:

- When piglets can eat and drink on their own
- When piglets demonstrate independence
- When piglets are not entirely reliant on their mother sow
- All of the above are signs that your piglet is ready to wean. Depending on the breed, this could range from 4 to 8 weeks of age. Wean the most independent and largest sized piglets first, preferably before the 4 week mark, if you have a sow that has been badly depleted by a large litter. The only exception is if you believe it is vital for the health/survival of the sow.

Tips for better weaning

Introduce food pre-weaning: When it's time to wean the piglets, providing dry creep feed might help them adjust to the new diet. Three to five days before weaning, put one and a half to two and a half pounds of dry feed in their crates. Pick a food that has easily digestible components that tastes and smells like sow's milk.

Keep Similar Feeds: Throughout the weaning phase, it is vital to continue giving your piglets a comparable beginning meal. Choose beginning feed that tastes comparable to the creep feed you introduced to thc piglets. Taste is really important to piglets. To return to the feeder, they must appreciate what they are eating.

Provide Fresh Feed: Put fresh feed in feeders and carefully on mats. Pigs prefer to eat in groups, so create a group eating routine to encourage them to eat throughout the day. Ensure that fresh feed is available all day and that the pig can easily discover the mats, feeders, and water.

Manure disposal

In the morning and evening, dry solid manure can be collected and stored in the dung shed. In settling tanks, the liquid fraction of urine and washings can be disposed of. Pigs can be effectively integrated into a biogas plant to meet the cooking and lighting demands of farmers. It can also be integrated into agriculture and fish culture, increasing the overall economic efficiency of the system. Pig dung, whether dried or composted, makes excellent organic manure.

15

Pig Diseases

Identification of Diseased Animals

Detection of compromised pigs necessitates awareness and fast decisions about treatment, transportation, and/or culling.

Walking the pens daily to observe the pigs will aid in the early identification of healthy and unwell pigs. Before unsettling a group of pigs, try to assess them from afar. This allows you to assess their behaviour.

Check the pens for down or lame animals, watch for increased activity around the water or feeders, and listen for coughing or sneezing. Inspect the ventilation system for improper or poorly managed air quality.

Then, enter the pen area quietly and study the pigs individually utilising B.E.S.T. Method. This acronym stands for:

- Body
- Eyes/Ears/Nose
- Skin/Hair-coat
- Temperament.

In a consistent and systematic routine, observe each pig, in a clockwise direction, from snout to tail (over the back) and then tail to snout (across and under the belly).

The body should be robust and sturdy. The spine, hips, and ribs should not be visible in nursery or finishing pigs. Prominent spines indicate malnutrition or malabsorption. The tail is free of lesions and/or bites, and there is no diarrhoea in the area around the anus and vulva. The pig's feet and legs appear to be identical, with no swelling, sores, or cracks on the toes, and it appears that the pig can walk normally. The pig appears to have a full stomach. Panting, thumping/laboured breathing, coughing, wheezing, or sneezing are not signs of a healthy pig. Atypical behaviour includes shaking, lying prostrate, paddling, and losing balance.

Pink skin around the eyes, ears, and nose should be clear of sores and secretions. A sick pig's eyes may be dull, sunken, or inflamed. Cloudy or dark discharge around the eye is common in conditions of respiratory disease. Pig ears should be clean and free of accumulations, swelling, parasites, and injury. The nose should be cool and moist, and devoid of lesions.

Smooth, clean, and firmly packed skin and hair are ideal. Parasites, disease, conflict, or nutritional deficiency can all create lumps, blisters, scaly or hair loss, or crustiness. Skin scales or crusting could indicate mange.

Temperament: Pigs are naturally curious and should react to their surroundings with genuine interest. When approached, pigs may move away, but they may return and investigate, snuffling and gnawing at boots and clothing. Sick pigs may have their heads and ears down, avoiding you and moving away from the group.

To summarise, good pig care entails identifying sick animals and acting quickly to treat, cull, or euthanize the sick pig. The first step in identifying a sick pig is to observe all of the pigs in a pen or area as a population, followed by clockwise individual pig observations. When employing the B.E.S.T. strategy, the stockperson will remember to observe all of the pig's features. Everyone who works with pigs must be able to recognise the symptoms of common diseases.

Classical swine fever

Pigs of any age can be affected by this disease. High death rates. Conjunctivitis, high fever, and profuse discharge from the eyes and nose are the main clinical manifestations. If you suspect it is affecting your herd, notify your veterinarian and local authorities.

CSF is one of the world's most economically destructive pandemic viral pig illnesses. Many governments take it very seriously and implement stringent control strategies, such as mandatory vaccination or killing, as well as eradication policies.

Almost all of the pigs in a vulnerable (unvaccinated) herd are afflicted. Fever, malaise, lack of appetite, diarrhoea, paralysis, miscarriage, mummification, and the birth of trembling piglets are all symptoms of the virus. The death rate is high.

Attenuated vaccinations are highly effective. It also does not spread through the wind, insects, or birds, so conventional agricultural biosecurity efforts should keep it out. It does, however, persist in raw and cured meat, which should not be fed to pigs.

Clinical signs

The pathogenicity of the virus that causes CSF varies. Some strains are extremely virulent and cause severe disease in a short period of time. Some strains are low virulent and induce chronic (long-term) sickness, whereas others are intermediate and cause subacute disease.

Acute disease

- Clinical indications usually occur first in a small percentage of growing pigs who exhibit non-specific signs of depression, drowsiness, and aversion to getting up or eating. If you wake them awake, they may come to the feeder but eat very little or nothing before returning to lie down. Their heads are low and their tails are limp as they stroll and stand. These symptoms worsen over time, and more pigs are affected.
- Younger piglets may appear chilly, quiver, and huddle together.
- Affected pigs may appear constipated at first, but this usually develops to yellow-grey diarrhoea as the disease progresses. Some pigs may develop conjunctivitis (inflammation of the eye surface) with thin secretions early on. This worsens over time, with the discharge thickening until some of the eyelids are totally closed and glued.
- A high temperature of more than 42°C (107°F) is a consistent early symptom that lasts throughout the disease until just before death. Check the rectal temperatures of the sick pigs. If they are all high, CSF is a strong possibility.

As the disease advances, the infected pigs become very thin and fragile, with a stumbling gait. This is most likely due to weakness at first, but it is later related to infection and damage to the spinal nerves. A drunken walk and a tendency to tumble into a seated or laying position come from partial paralysis of the hind end. The pigs' diarrhoea worsens, and some vomit yellowish bile. The pigs' skin turns purple, beginning with the ears and tail and progressing to the nose, lower legs, belly, and back. Pigs that are infected die after 10-20 days. Some pigs have convulsions before they die.

Sub-acute disease

The early signs in growing pigs are alike but they progress more gradually and are less severe. Affected pigs may be ill for up to 30 days before they die.

Chronic infection

- The virus has the ability to cross the placenta and infect piglets in the sow's uterus. Sows that have not been fully vaccinated and become infected, or sows that become infected with a low virulence virus, may appear normal but give birth to trembling piglets, many of whom die.

- If the virus penetrates the placenta before the piglets' immune systems have matured, they may be born seemingly healthy, but weak, and may go on to be persistent carriers without first exhibiting clinical indications. They shed virus and pose a threat to other pigs. They may show normal clinical indications at several weeks or months of age, although they are likely to be milder, last longer, and lack high temperatures.
- A virus that infects piglets in the uterus may cause death, mummification, miscarriage, or the birth of frail piglets. Vaccinating pregnant sows with some of the attenuated virus vaccines resulted in trans-placental infection of unborn piglets, with comparable negative outcomes. It is stated that the newer attenuated vaccinations are safer.
- Low virulence variants of the virus may also grow in the reproductive tracts of unprotected or partially vaccinated boars. The vaccination virus itself was considered to achieve this in some older attenuated vaccines, resulting in returns to service and miscarriages.

Diagnosis

- A diagnosis can be made in acute or subacute epidemics based on the characteristic clinical signs and post-mortem lesions; however African swine fever and Salmonella choleraesuis infection generate some comparable signs and lesions. Salmonella choleraesuis is frequently a co-infection with CSF virus, activated from a dormant condition by the CSF viral infection.
- Clinical symptoms and lesions are less diagnostic in chronic cases and may simply elicit a suspicion of CSF.
- Laboratory tests should be performed in all suspected instances to confirm the diagnosis.
- Sending complete dead pigs to the diagnostic laboratory allows pathologists to sample what they want. If just samples can be sent, tonsils are the greatest choice.
- Pig tonsils are really easy to locate. Remove the skin and flesh from beneath and between the lower jaw bone, including the tongue. The tonsils are two enormous red patches, each around the size of the tip of your thumb or slightly larger. Send them packed with ice rather than frozen.
- Viruses are found all over the body. In addition to the tonsils, the spleen, kidneys, and the last few inches of the small intestine are the ideal organs to send.

Post-mortem

- Post-mortem examination findings are normally interpreted by a qualified individual, but in the case of CSF, a skilled pig person should be able to recognise some of the more obvious pathologies.
- The image is remarkable when pigs are lay on their backs after death and opened up for examination. Small haemorrhages are common throughout the body, with greater haemorrhages in some organs such as lymph nodes. Some of these may be brilliant red and blood-filled. Larger haemorrhages may also occur in the lungs and beneath the skin.
- The kidney surfaces are frequently characterised as looking like speckled duck eggs, with varying sized bleeding patches.
- There may be dark elevated patches of dead tissue on the spleen. Similar patches of dead tissue can be found in other organs (for example, the tonsils), although they are more difficult to locate.
- Severe pneumonia, bleeding, and pleurisy in the lungs are common complications of secondary bacterial infection.
- Except for a small amount of brilliantly coloured liquid, the stomach and gut are normally empty. Raised 'button ulcers' on the inner lining of the large intestine near its confluence with the small intestine are unusual lesions to watch for.

Prevention

Vaccination

- Routine immunisation is practised and may be mandatory in enzootic and high risk areas. Inactivated vaccinations were widely used, although they occasionally contained live virus, resulting in illness. Live attenuated vaccinations, the most modern of which are relatively safe and efficacious, have essentially superseded inactivated vaccines. Pigs develop protective immunity within a week to ten days of immunisation, and the protection lasts for two to three years (i.e. the lifetime of many sows and boars). Piglets suckled by vaccinated sows acquire colostral protection that lasts around 6-8 weeks. They cannot be successfully vaccinated at this time because maternal antibodies neutralise the vaccine virus before it has had opportunity to promote immunity.
- CSF virus has only one mutationally stable serotype that causes significant long-lasting protection. The virus in CSF vaccinations was attenuated by repeated passage in rabbits (referred to as 'lapinised vaccines' or 'Chinese strain vaccines'). These are still accessible in some parts of the world,

but many vaccinations today contain viruses that have been attenuated by continuous cell culture growth.

- In a defined area where the CSF virus is endemic, it is common practise to first vaccine all pigs above the age of two weeks. Piglets delivered to vaccinated sows would be immunised at the age of 8 weeks. This policy frequently results in the pathogen being eradicated from that area.

On-farm precautions

- If you farm in a place where CSF is prevalent or where there is a risk of CSF, consider vaccinating your herd on a regular basis if immunisation is permitted. This drastically reduces the likelihood of contamination.
- CSF virus does not spread as quickly as other viruses (e.g. TGE and FMD). It is not windborne, unlike FMD. As a result, the careful application of simple biosecurity measures should keep it out of the herd.
- If CSF is present in your area, critical precautions include limiting visitors, taking precautions against vehicle contamination, and not letting pig meat products near any pigs.
- Any replacement pigs brought onto the premises should be quarantined and originate from known safe suppliers. The disease has become relatively mild in some locations, and its spread may go unnoticed.

Stray animals, particularly wild pigs and boars, should be kept away from pig structures.

Treatment

There is no treatment.

African swine fever (ASF)

Pigs of any age can be affected by this disease. There is a significant rate of fatality. The main clinical signs include blue-purple cyanosis of the snout, ears, tail, and lower legs, a high fever, and a lot of discharge from the eyes and nose. African swine fever is caused by the *Asfarviridae* family of viruses which are different from the viruses associated with Classical swine fever.

African swine fever (ASF) is so similar to classical swine fever (CSF) (hog cholera) that laboratory tests are required to tell them apart. The clinical symptoms and post-mortem lesions of the two diseases are virtually identical. ASF is caused by a separate virus that is distinct from CSF and exclusively infects domestic and wild pigs as well as a variety of soft ticks. The virus is found in warthogs and bush pigs in Africa south of the equator, although infection causes no clinical disease. It spreads between warthogs and the soft-bodied ticks that live in their burrows. It is transmitted and perpetuated by ticks at all phases of their life cycle. It is also found in some African countries' domestic pigs.

The pig is the only natural host of the viruses, which means the virus does not harm people or other animals. This is not to say that people and other animals cannot transfer the virus as carriers; African swine fever (ASF) is widely conveyed by arthropods, such as the soft-bodied tick, by blood sucling from infected pigs.

Contamination usually occurs by direct contact with infected or carrier pig tissue and bodily fluids, such as discharges from the nose, mouth, urine, and faeces, or contaminated sperm. It also spreads through the transportation and consumption of infected food products, and some cases have resulted from failing to meet biosecurity rules by feeding waste food to domestic pigs. A highly virulent strain of ASF is thought to have been introduced to farmed pigs and, later, wild boar populations.

Although the virus does not cause disease in wild boar and hogs, it is highly communicable across all swine species and can live in pigs for long periods of time after slaughter, even in frozen carcasses. It's also worth noting that curing and smoking pork products don't kill the virus.

It is critical to identify the disease that is infecting a herd as soon as possible; ASF and classical swine fever are caused by viruses that can only be distinguished by laboratory testing. Notifying a veterinarian as soon as any symptoms appear is the best way to ensure proper quarantine and treatment protocols are followed - it could save the rest of your pigs.

Clinical signs

- High fever 40-42°C.
- Loss of hunger.
- Depression.
- Lethargic
- Very shaky when stood up.
- Vomiting and diarrhoea with bloody discharge.
- Extremities become cyanotic.
- Discrete haemorrhages appear in the skin mainly on the ears and flanks.
- Animals huddle together and generally shivering.

- Abnormal breathing.
- Heavy discharge from eyes and nose.
- Comatose state and death within a few days.
- May show conjunctivitis with reddening of the conjunctival mucosa and ocular discharges.
- Pregnant sows usually undergo miscarriage or deliver stillborn piglets.

Because the mortality rate in infected groups of pigs is significant and there is no vaccine shown to prevent or cure infection, it is critical that management begin on the farm. Infected countries in Europe, South America, and the Caribbean have implemented a slaughter policy in order to remove the virus from the herd. Mild variants of the virus also exist, causing a weaker but equally deadly disease in domestic pig herds; individuals from these herds must be destroyed as well to prevent pathogenesis.

Diagnosis

Pigs that die early in an epidemic may not have visible lesions, but as the disease spreads, the lesions become more visible. Bright crimson haemorrhages in the lymph nodes, kidneys, heart, and body cavity linings are common findings. Excess haemorrhagic fluid and gelatinous fluid in the lungs are other possibilities. On gentle pressure, the spleen may expand, discolour, and collapse.

The veterinarian will need to send samples to a laboratory that specialises in diagnosing CSF and ASF. Blood, lymph nodes, spleen, and, in chronic instances, serum for serology are the best samples to send. If it is CSF rather than ASF, the tonsils may also be sent. Pig tonsils are really easy to locate. Cut the skin and flesh under and between the lower jaw bone and tongue of the deceased pig while it was lying on its back. The tonsils are two enormous red patches, each around the size of the tip of your thumb or slightly larger. Small holes or depressions cover their surfaces.

Primary cultures of pig bone marrow or peripheral blood leucocytes can be used to isolate the virus. Fluorescent antibody assays can also identify virus in infected cells. Antibodies are also detected using ELISA assays. Samples can be injected into experimental pigs in dubious instances. Porcine dermatitis and nephropathy syndrome, which occur on occasion in most pig producing locations, can clinically and post-mortem resembles ASF and CSF. A laboratory check may be required to rule them out of the diagnosis.

Transmission

- Bites from soft-bodied ticks, lice, and flies; Feeding of contaminated feed and contaminated food waste used to augment feed;
- Contaminated needles and surgical equipment were used, and infected pigs were introduced into the herd.
- Within the herd, the virus is primarily transmitted through direct contact with infected bodily secretions, faeces, and vomit.

Prevention

- There is no live or attenuated vaccine for the prevention of ASF therefore control of the virus is reliant on strict biosecurity.
- Do not feed food waste to domestic pigs; do not leave food waste accessible for wild swine species to access.
- Adhere to strict biosecurity guidelines. Bring no pig meat into farms, and keep all meals to a canteen. Before and after interaction with pigs, all farm personnel should be taught in hand and equipment sanitization.
- Make certain that no wild pigs or products polluted by such wild species come into touch with domestic pigs.
- People should be counselled and informed about the dangers of bringing pork products from affected areas.

Treatment

There is no treatment.

All infected animals must be isolated and culled immediately upon confirmation of presence of the virus.

Foot and mouth disease (FMD)

All age group pigs are susceptible to this disease. The main clinical indications include lameness, vesicles, and blisters, as well as salivating pigs. If you suspect it is affecting your herd, notify your veterinarian and local authorities. If sudden widespread lameness arises, this disease should always be considered. The greatest significant impediment to international trading in animals and animal products is FMD. As a result, enormous sums of money have been invested on control and eradication programmes, as well as research. As a result, the FMD virus is better understood than nearly any other animal infection.

Infected pigs can expel massive amounts of infective virus as aerosols. The aerosol virus is rapidly inactivated in dry weather when there are high temperature, therefore the wind does not carry infective aerosols very far. In humid cloudy weather with a persistent light wind blowing across flat farmland, an infective virus may survive long enough to infect additional herds up to 60 kilometres away. Infective virus has been demonstrated to travel up to 300km over water under the same climatic conditions, therefore locating your pig herd on an island in a lake will not stop it. Windborne illness is impossible to avoid. Even if your pigs are housed in a closed structure, the aerosol virus can enter through the ventilation system and you may bring it in on your boots or clothes from outside.

Clinical signs

- Sudden prevalent lameness.
- High salivation.
- Vesicles are evident on the skin. Common sites are: top of the claws;
- heels; nose; tongue; lips; teats of recently farrowed sows.
- Within 24 hours numerous of the vesicles will burst.
- Chomping of jaws.
- Inappetence.
- Depression.
- Fever of about 40.5°C (105°F).
- Thimbling (complete loss of hooves).
- Abortion in sows.
- Death in severe cases.
- Increased morality in piglet

Prevention

- In high risk areas regular vaccination may be practised mainly to protect the breeding stock.
- Ring vaccination may be used around the affected region.
- If you farm in an FMD-risk area, you should take extra care to protect your herd from infection. If you have a herd of cattle, goats, sheep, or pigs, you should take preventative measures and keep an eye out for the appearance of usual clinical indications.
- Basic biosecurity measures are vital in helping to reduce the spread of disease.

- Only allow necessary visitors on the farm, and bring your own boots and clothing.
- If visitors do not shower, make sure their hands are washed.
- As far as possible, restrict people's movement between buildings.
- Install foot dips at all service and feed delivery stations. Apply an authorised disinfectant at the proper dilution.
- Go over all cleaning and disinfection processes again. Only allow vehicles that have been washed and disinfected to visit your farm.
- Take extra measures when using loading ramps. Provide specific boots and overalls for usage solely on the loading ramp. Before and after usage, disinfect all loading areas. Ensure that drainage is directed away from the farm.
- Clean all pens carefully. These should be disinfected and dried between pig groups.

Treatment

There is no treatment. Animals should be culled.

Swine Pox

This is a virus-borne disease caused by the swine pox virus, which can persist outside of the pig for extended periods of time and is resistant to environmental changes. It is a vesicular condition with little circular red patches 10-20mm in diameter that begin with a vesicle holding straw-colored fluid in the centre. After two to three days, the vesicle ruptures, forming a scab that eventually turns black. The lesions can appear everywhere on the body, but they are most common around the flanks, abdomens, and occasionally the ears. The condition normally resolves itself on its own within three weeks. It is similar to greasy pig illness, pustular dermatitis, and the allergic type of mange. Close examination shows swine pox lesions.

Clinical signs

Little spherical red patches 10-20mm in diameter, beginning with a vesicle filled with straw-colored fluid in the centre.

After two to three days, the vesicle ruptures, forming a scab that gradually turns black.

Secondary dermatitis is possible.

Transmission

- It can be spread by lice or mange mites.
- Skin abrasions.
- Fighting and mixing of pigs.

Control

Control of swine pox is based on herd immunity and avoidance of transmission. Pox is rarely a problem if the usual virus vectors, particularly hog lice, are managed with insecticides or eradication. Congenital swine pox is usually a sporadic, self-limiting condition. There are no therapies.

Porcine parvovirus (PPV)

Porcine parvovirus (PPV) infection is a common and serious cause of infectious infertility. PPV is a strong virus that replicates regularly in the intestine of the pig without causing clinical symptoms and is found in pig populations all over the world. In the stillbirth mummification embryonic death and infertility (SMEDI) condition, PPV is one of the viruses involved.

It is almost certain to be present in larger herds and is an infection that must be lived with and managed rather than eradicated. It may or may not have died out in smaller herds with a previously PPV positive pig.

Most viruses do not survive outside of the host for long periods of time; however, PPV is remarkable in that it can survive in the environment for many months and is resistant to most disinfectants; the most likely reason for this is that it is widespread and difficult to eradicate.

PPV is not harmful to human or other agricultural animals, and it poses no concern to food safety.

Clinical signs

In acute outbreaks of the disease, the infection causes no clinical indications other than the existence of mummified piglets ranging in size from 3 to 16 cm at farrowing. PPV spreads slowly from foetus to foetus inside the womb, therefore the sizes of mummified pigs will vary throughout the litter, and depending on the gestation age when the sow became infected, some may survive.

Other indicative observations are:

- There has been an increase in the number of stillbirths. They are related to the farrowing process being delayed due to the presence of mummified piglets.

- Embryonic loss before 35 days of gestation has been associated to small litters.
- There has been an increase in low birth weight piglets, but no increase in neonatal mortality.
- The afterbirth contains little mummified pigs.
- Abortions caused by PPV are uncommon.
- Sporadic cases within a herd are typically restricted to newly purchased naive gilts or sows.
- Decreased vaccine efficacy in gilts because maternal immunity in live piglets can survive up to 7 months but only in a few gilts, interfering with vaccine response.
- Up to 50% of gilts in larger sero-positive herds may be sero-negative after mating. There were no more signs of sickness in the breeding females.
- In bigger herds with multiple farrowing, the acute sickness lasts about 2 months, then fades for a month, with subsequent instances of mummified piglets occurring for another month. It can take up to four months for PPV to infect all of the sows in an untreated herd. Such outbreaks are anticipated to occur every 3-4 years in non-vaccinated herds as viral circulation lower and high. A vulnerable population eventually emerges during periods of few or no PPV cases.
- Surprisingly, sows with total foetal loss can have a pseudo-pregnancy. In other circumstances, the sow reaches farrowing with normal udder development, even to the point of producing milk, yet no live births occur. In this case, a prostaglandin injection is required to initiate farrowing, which eject the mummified piglets present inside the womb. These animals would not farrow otherwise since live foetuses are required to commence farrowing.

Predisposing factors

- The herd's immunological condition, i.e. lack of immunity, is the predisposing factor. Immunity will be present when PPV positive herds combine gilts before mating age with either PPV positive pigs or retain on land recently occupied by positive pigs. If the herd's breeding stock has previously recovered from PPV, they will be immune for the rest of their lives.
- In small herds, however, the PPV may die out, leaving the new gilts and sows susceptible. You must also assess whether the infection has entirely spread across the herd and whether you have pens of naive pigs.

- The most effective strategy to safeguard your herd is to vaccinate all stock, and failure to vaccinate, incorrect vaccination techniques, or improper storage can leave your herd vulnerable. Vaccinate boars as well, as they can shed the virus in their sperm.

Diagnosis

- PPV disease might be suspected in the absence of any other indicators of illness in the breeding females by increases in various sized (3 to 16 cm length) mummified pigs and small litter sizes.
- The mummified piglets can be studied in the lab for a laboratory diagnosis of a current infection in your herd using a Fluorescent Antibody Test - antibodies to PPV are labelled with a fluorescent dye that binds to tissue from the mummified piglets and glows under a UV light. Send little mummified pigs from small litters (less than 16 cm) to a laboratory for fluorescent antibody tests. These will determine whether or not the foetus perished as a result of PPV infection.
- Because many sows are positive and normal, serologically (searching for PPV antibodies in the serum) will not aid in the diagnosis of present disease. If the suspected PPV case is detected early, 'paired sera' can be collected a week apart to look for a dramatic increase in antibody levels.
- Blood screening all of the sows in a herd on one time only reveals the percentage of animals who have previously been exposed to PPV and which are vulnerable. When an animal is exposed to PPV, it becomes immune for the remainder of its life.

Prevention

Because PPV cannot be eradicated from a herd, the goal should be to manage and prevent acute cases. Routine vaccination of gilts and boars before to entering the breeding herd, along with yearly boosters for all pigs, should be adequate to protect the herd. However, studies have shown that if an infected breeding female has been vaccinated or has been exposed to PPV in the past, the immune system is quickly re-stimulated when exposed to PPV (within 5-7 days). This is enough to prevent sickness and stimulate long-term immunity.

If you have an unvaccinated herd and an acute epidemic occurs, vaccinate the breeding herd immediately to prevent infection in susceptible pigs. The initial dosage of vaccine takes 10 days to take action. The first dosage will activate the immune system and develop a low amount of antibody; the annual booster or exposure to PPV will typically be adequate to protect the unborn litter because infection takes 10-14 days to reach the placenta.

Treatment

There is no treatment.

Swine vesicular disease

Swine vesicular disease is a pig-borne viral vesicular illness caused by an enterovirus. It is useful as a differential diagnostic for foot-and-mouth disease, which is clinically indistinguishable from it. Swine vesicular disease (SVD) is a temporary pig disease characterised by vesicular sores on the hooves, nose, and mouth. SVD is usually mild, and it can infect pigs subclinically. It must be distinguished from foot-and-mouth disease (FMD), eradication is costly, and embargoes on pig and pork product exports are frequently imposed on nations not free of SVD. Pigs are considered the lone natural host of the virus, while it can infect sheep in close contact with infected pigs.

Signs and Symptoms

Fresh or healing vesicular lesions on the feet, particularly the coronary band, and, less frequently, other sites such as the mouth, lips, teats, or nose are the predominant clinical indicators of SVD. Lesions might be moderate or invisible, especially if the pigs are maintained on soft bedding. The lesions are comparable to those seen in FMD, swine vesicular exanthema, and vesicular stomatitis; however, infected pigs often do not lose condition, and the lesions heal quickly. Nervous system symptoms have been described, however they are rarely seen in the field.

Diagnosis

Laboratory testing of samples of epithelium, faeces, or serum from affected animals confirms the diagnosis of SVD. Antigen-detection ELISA, viral isolation, or reverse-transcriptase PCR assays are used to detect viruses. Serologic diagnosis is accomplished with the use of an antibody-detection ELISA or a virus neutralisation test; however, low specificity may be an issue, especially in older animals. In clinical circumstances, lesion material collected in phosphate-buffered saline is recommended. Subclinical infection can be detected using a reverse-transcriptase PCR assay or virus isolation on pen-floor faeces samples.

Control

Countries free of SVD can maintain their status by restricting pig and pork product imports or guaranteeing that pork products are treated (heat or otherwise) to eliminate the virus. Garbage feeding to pigs may be prohibited or regulated in order to assure full cooking of raw animal products. Any suspected epidemic should be notified to the proper authorities as soon as possible. If SVD does arise, it is controlled through biosecurity measures such as limiting pig mobility. Vaccines are not commercially available. To detect subclinically infected herds, extensive serosurveillance is required, and seroreactor herds must be followed up on with clinical inspection and faecal virus testing. Because the virus is exceedingly resistant in the environment and stable throughout a wide pH range, full disinfection of premises, trucks, and equipment is required. Strong alkalis are the most effective disinfectants, however hypochlorites or acid-containing iodophors can be employed when organic material is not present.

Pseudorabies

Pseudorabies is a viral disease that is widespread throughout the world. The major host is swine, however other species are occasionally affected. In growing pigs, clinical indicators include reproductive failure as well as CNS and respiratory abnormalities. Clinical indicators are used to make the diagnosis, which is then validated by serology, PCR, or viral isolation. Although no specific treatment is available, highly effective vaccinations are available.

Signs and symptoms

The clinical indications of the pseudorabies virus in pigs vary according to the age of the infected animal. Young pigs are more vulnerable, with losses reaching 100% in 7-day-old piglets. In general, signs of CNS disease (eg, tremors and paddling) are seen. If weaned pigs become infected, pulmonary illness is the predominant clinical concern, especially if additional bacterial infections are present. Pseudorabies virus has been shown to disrupt the activity of alveolar macrophages, limiting these cells' ability to digest and eliminate germs.

Infected pigs of all ages exhibit a widespread feverish reaction, anorexia, and weight loss. Mortality in grower and finisher pigs can be quite low, but it can approach 50% in piglets. Sneezing and dyspnea are common, and CNS involvement has been recorded on occasion. In nonporcine species like cats, dogs, cattle, and small ruminants, clinical indicators include sudden death, strong local itching, CNS indications (circling, manic behaviour, paralysis), fever, and respiratory distress.

Lesions

Gross lesions caused by pseudorabies virus infection are frequently undetected. It is possible to have serous rhinitis, necrotic tonsils, or hemorrhagic pulmonary lymph nodes. There may be pulmonary edoema as well as pneumonic lesions of secondary bacterial infections. Necrotic foci (2-3 mm in diameter) can be found all over the liver. These lesions are most commonly encountered in young (less than 7 days old) piglets.

Diagnosis

Other diagnostic techniques for identifying pseudorabies virus, in addition to visual and microscopic abnormalities, include virus isolation, PCR fluorescent antibody testing, and serologic testing. The organs of choice for viral isolation include the brain, spleen, and lung. Virus isolation from acutely infected animals can be accomplished using nasal swabs. To inhibit bacterial development, nose specimens must be maintained and transported in cold, sterile saline containing antibiotics. The fluorescent antibody test can be done on either the tonsil or the brain.

Control and Treatment

Although there is no specific treatment for acute pseudorabies virus infection, immunisation can reduce clinical indications in certain pigs. It is common practise to advocate bulk vaccination of all pigs on the farm using a modified-live virus vaccine. Intranasal immunisation of sows and neonatal piglets aged 1-7 days, followed by intramuscular vaccination of all other pigs on the premises, reduces virus shedding and improves survival. It is suggested that breeding herds be vaccinated quarterly, and finisher pigs be immunised when maternal antibody levels have decreased. Regular immunisation resulted in great disease control. To manage secondary bacterial infections, concurrent antibiotic therapy via feed and IM injection is indicated.

Pleuropneumonia

Pleuropneumonia, a dangerous respiratory infection, is caused by Actinobacillus pleuropneumoniae. Clinical indicators include fever, anorexia, inability to move, breathing difficulties, and sudden death. The diagnosis is confirmed by bacterial culture. Although antibiotics can be used to treat sick animals, control is achieved by removing pathogens at the breeding stock level.

Pleuropneumonia is a severe and contagious respiratory disease that primarily affects young pigs, however adults may be affected in the early stages of an outbreak. It has a short course, a fast onset, and a high morbidity and fatality rate. It is found all across the world yet, some studies suggest that severity is decreasing in areas where it has been established for a long period.

Clinical Findings

Pleuropneumonia occurs unexpectedly and spreads swiftly in previously uninfected herds. In the absence of clinical indications, some pigs may be found dead. There are "thumps" and open-mouth breathing, as well as blood-stained, frothy nasal and oral discharge. Common symptoms include a fever of up to 107°F, anorexia, and aversion to movement.

A pleuropneumoniae infection, despite being mostly a disease of growing pigs, can kill individuals or cause sows to miscarry. The condition can grow from acute to chronic. In untreated cases, morbidity can approach 50%, and death is severe. Survivors often grow at a slower rate and have a persistent cough.

Possible outcomes include deaths in transportation and carcass condemnation. Infections with mycoplasma, pasteurellae, porcine reproductive and respiratory illness, or swine influenza virus are common.

Treatment and Control

Pleuropneumonia is difficult to treat since it develops quickly and persists in infected herds. Ceftiofur, tilmicosin, tetracyclines, synthetic penicillins, tylosin, and sulfonamides have all been utilised. The first treatment should be parenteral, followed by medication given as water or feed, which may help protect contact pigs.

Lower stocking rates and greater ventilation are indicated for preventive, all in/all out management. Replacements from pleuropneumoniae-free herds in disease-free herds should be purchased; if the disease proves difficult to treat, herd depopulation and repopulation should be considered. Due to breeding stock removal methods, pleuropneumonia is rarely encountered in today's modern confinement swine production systems.

Mycoplasmal pneumonia

Mycoplasma hyopneumoniae is a prevalent cause of pneumonia in pigs across the world. It also frequently results in subclinical infection, which produces post-mortem lung lesions. Clinical indicators, if present, include a dry cough and decreased growth. Clinical indicators, distinctive lesions, and confirmation by PCR assay can all be used to make a diagnosis. Improved management methods, antibiotic treatment, and immunisation can all help to control some diseases.

Mycoplasmal pneumonia is an infectious pig pneumonia that is persistent and usually mild. A prolonged dry cough, poor growth, intermittent flares of overt respiratory distress, and a high prevalence of lung lesions in killed pigs are all symptoms of the condition. It spreads globally and becomes endemic in affected herds.

Clinical epidemics of mycoplasmal pneumonia might have a negative impact on growth rate and feed conversion. The disease's effects are unequal and unpredictable, limiting the efficiency and flexibility of large manufacturing units. Mycoplasmal pneumonia may remain essentially asymptomatic in swine operations that have strong disease control strategies in place. However, pathogen eradication appears to be the only way to accomplish absolute disease control.

Mycoplasmal pneumonia is also known as enzootic pneumonia, a disease state caused predominantly by M hyopneumoniae. Pigs of all ages are susceptible; transmission to suckling piglets can occur from sows of all parities, but first-parity (gilt) litters are the most common. The disease's onset may be most visible in the final stage about 18-20 weeks of age.

Clinical Findings

The most prevalent symptom of mycoplasmal pneumonia is nonproductive coughing, which is particularly noticeable when pigs are roused. Morbidity is considerable in endemically infected herds, although clinical symptoms are limited and mortality is low. Commonly impacted production indicators include average daily weight increase and days to market weight.

Individual pigs or groups of pigs acquire severe pneumonia on a sporadic basis. Season and other pressures such as transitory virus illnesses, parasite migration, and mingling pigs are common predisposing factors. When the disease first enters a naive herd, it is frequently more severe.

Lesions

On physical examination, damaged lungs are grey or purple, with consolidated regions most typically in the apical and cardiac lobes. Old lesions are easily distinguished and gradually heal, leaving obvious scars. The lymph nodes may swell. Histologically, the bronchioles have inflammatory cells, perivascular and peribronchiolar cuffing, and significant lymphoid hyperplasia.

Diagnosis

Mycoplasmal pneumonia is frequently suspected based on clinical, histopathologic, and herd epidemiologic data. M hyopneumoniae can be seen in impression smears of the damaged lung's sliced surface, recognised using a fluorescent antibody method or in situ hybridization, and isolated and identified in culture. The aforementioned laboratory tests, however, are not frequently conducted by practising veterinarians.

Control

Improvements in housing and husbandry, notably ventilation and space allowed, can lessen the economic impact of mycoplasmal pneumonia in pigs. The "all-in/all-out" management of pigs from birth to market is particularly effective in reducing illness effects; this method improves growth performance and lowers lung lesions. Commercially available inactivated mycoplasmal bacterins are adjuvanted whole-cell preparations. Bacterins protect growing pigs from the development of gross lesions and greatly reduce clinical symptoms (coughing). Vaccination, on the other hand, does not prevent infection.

When Mycoplasma spp. enters a herd, mass treatment with antibiotics effective against Mycoplasma spp. helps to minimise the severity of symptoms. When illness outbreaks occur in endemic herds, treating individual pigs with antimicrobials frequently results in remission, presumably through secondary bacterial control. Starting with mycoplasmal pneumonia-free foundation stock and taking stringent safeguards against direct and indirect contact with pigs from other herds is recommended.

Porcine Proliferative Enteritis

Porcine proliferative enteritis (PPE) is an intestinal condition characterised by crypt enterocyte proliferation, inflammation, and, in certain cases, ulceration or haemorrhage. The mucous membrane of a portion of the small and/or large intestine is invariably thickened in lesions. Lesions vary greatly in terms of location, extent, and longevity.

Clinical signs

There has been uncertainty related to nomenclature, lesions, and clinical signs of PPE, mainly due to the difference that exists in clinical signs, age of pig affected, and gross lesions. In addition, a syndrome (hemorrhagic bowel syndrome or HBS) of unexpected death with blood in the intestinal tract is often puzzled with this condition. Acute PPE instances are most commonly seen in late finishing pigs and young breeding swine. Acute diarrhoea, paleness, weakness, and fast mortality are typical; lesions include mucosal growth and bleeding. Subacute to chronic instances are more common in the grower stages, manifesting as intermittent diarrhoea, wasting, and growth rate fluctuation; lesions typically contain necrotic enteritis and can be easily confused with salmonellosis. Morbidity and mortality are varying with either presentation. Some pigs may have significant mucosal proliferation in the terminal small intestine but be clinically asymptomatic.

Diagnosis

A cautious diagnosis frequently can be made on the basis of clinical signs along with the presence of characteristic gross and microscopic lesions, even though some cases of porcine circovirus type 2 (PCV2) enteritis can present themselves clinically very similar to PPE.

Control

To manage and treat PPE, various antibiotics are frequently provided to feed for several weeks during or after periods of stress and outbreaks. Tylosin, tetracyclines, lincomycin, tiamulin, and carbadox can be used to regulate experimental PPE. Various treatment techniques, including as pulse dosing and continuous medication, have been tried. Medication failures are common in breeding stock where animals are not fed ad libitum and hence get subtherapeutic doses of otherwise effective antimicrobials. PPE control has been a primary driver of the use of feed-grade antimicrobials in grow-finish swine.

When delivered appropriately via water or orally, an avirulent live vaccination appears to have extremely good effectiveness. Acclimatization vaccination of growing pigs and breeding gilts has been very successful in decreasing or eradicating clinical indications of PPE. Vaccination has allowed the elimination of ongoing administration of feed-grade antimicrobials in some herds.

Diarrhoea or Swine scour

Diarrhoea is the most prevalent and perhaps the most serious illness in sucking piglets. It is responsible for significant morbidity and mortality in some epidemics. In a well-managed herd, less than 3% of litters should require treatment at any given time, and piglet mortality from diarrhoea should be less than 0.5%. In severe outbreaks, mortality rates can reach 7% or more, and in individual untreated litters, they can reach 100%. E. coli and clostridia are the most common bacterial causes, and coccidia are the most common parasite.

The antibodies obtained passively from colostrum and milk is limited and might be overpowered by high levels of microorganisms in the environment. The greater the number of organisms consumed, the higher the danger of sickness. Environmental stress, like as freezing, also plays a role since it diminishes the resilience of the piglets. Thus, there is a delicate balance between the level of antibody on one hand and the weight of infection and stress on the other.

Clinical signs

Piglets

In acute disease:

- Previously good pig found dead.
- Huddle together, trembling or lie in a corner.
- The skin just about the rectum and tail is wet.
- Watery scour - distinctive smell.
- Vomiting.

As the diarrhoea progresses:

- Dehydrated.
- Sunken eyes.
- Leathery skin.

In sub-acute disease:

- Signs are alike but the effects on the piglet are less remarkable, more extended and mortality tends to be lower.
- This type of scour is frequently seen between 7 to 14 days of age.

Weaners

- The earliest symptoms are frequently mild fatigue, dehydration, and watery diarrhoea.
- In certain situations, blood or black tarry faeces may be visible, or they may appear as a paste with a variety of colours such as grey, white, yellow, and green.
- Pigs are wasteful and hairy.
- Sunken pupils.
- Dehydration causes fast weight loss.
- Pigs with sunken eyes and minor blueing of the extremities may be discovered dead.
- Good pigs may be discovered dead with no visible indications.
- Vomiting on occasion.

Diagnosis

When making a diagnosis, the big picture must be evaluated. TGE, epidemic diarrhoea, or PRRS are all possibilities for sudden outbreaks of scour involving huge numbers of litters with acute diarrhoea and significant mortality. It is always helpful in distinguishing these infections to know whether or not the herd has previously been exposed to any of these diseases. If this is first time being exposed, the outbreak is likely to be explosive.

Rotavirus diarrhoea typically emerges in waves in individual litters or groups of litters during the second part of breastfeeding. Coccidiosis has a 6-day incubation period and is typically associated with diarrhoea complexes ranging in age from 7 to 14 days. E. coli with acute diarrhoea is the most common cause at less than 5 days of age, especially in gilts' litters because they pass on lower levels of immunity. Clostridial infections can arise at this age as well.

Clinical examinations, therapeutic response (viral infections do not react to treatment), and laboratory investigation of the scour are used to make a diagnosis. Send a rectal swab or a live pig to the lab for culture analysis and antibiotic sensitivity testing.

Causes

Sows and piglets

- Inadequate pen floors.
- Poor pen hygiene as a result of poor drainage.
- Inadequate hygiene precautions between pens.
- Environmental pollution from one pen to the next, such as boots, brushes, shovels, clothing, and so on.
- Consistent usage of pens.
- Bacterial proliferation thrives under conditions of moisture, warmth, waste food, and faeces.
- The regular use of milk substitutes, especially if they get stale or contaminated, may increase the prevalence.
- Scour is more prevalent in large litters. This could be related to:
- Inadequate colostrum.
- Inadequate teat access.
- Inadequate crate design.
- Agalactia in the suckling.

Weaners and growers

Pre-weaning

- Consider the type, frequency and age of introduction of creep ration.
- Stop creep feeding previous to weaning and evaluate the effects.

At weaning

- Stress.
- Stocking density
- House temperatures
- Poor house hygiene.
- Water shortage.
- Feed type: Meal or pellets, wet or dry.
- Feeding practices.
- Quality of nutrition.

After weaning

- Air flow.
- Temperature fluctuations.
- High humidity.
- Creep feed management.
- Other diseases
- Age and weight at weaning.
- Floor surfaces

Prevention

- Between pens, disinfect the boots.
- When treating piglets, wear a disposable plastic apron to avoid significant contamination of clothing.
- After handling scrubbed litter, wash your hands.
- Brushes and shovels should be disinfected between uses.
- Ensure that farrowing houses are only utilised all-in, all-out, with a pressure wash and disinfection between batches.
- Before the house can be repopulated, the farrowing pens must be dry. Remember that moisture, warmth, discarded food, and faeces are all great conditions for bacterial growth.

- Pen floors should be kept in good condition. Scour is predisposed to by poor pen cleanliness combined with poor drainage.
- Examine the area of the pen floor where there are piglet faeces attentively. Is this a clogged drain? Do huge wet areas form? If so, cover them on a daily basis and remove them. This is a critical part of control.
- Check for leaks in nipple drinkers and feeding troughs.
- If the floors are slatted, ensure that faeces are removed daily from behind the sow from the day she enters the farrowing crates until at least 7 days post-farrowing. Also, if the floors are solid concrete, remove them every day throughout lactation.
- Keep creep habitats warm and comfortable at all times. Fluctuating temperatures are a crucial trigger factor to scour particularly from 7 to 14 days of life.
- Do not withhold on your heating costs. Many incidents of scour are caused by initiatives to reduce energy expenditures.
- Examine for excessive air flow and draughts. They are prone to scour.
- Consider getting an E. coli vaccine. Vaccines against E. coli only protect the piglet for the first 5 to 7 days of life.
- Examine the overall surroundings of the farrowing house. Bacterial growth is enhanced in poor conditions, and a much higher bacterial challenge is likely to tear down the colostral immunity.
- Examine the sow's health. Animals suffering from enteric or respiratory disease, lameness, or mastitis are more likely to scour the litter.
- If at all feasible, avoid using milk substitutes. Their regular usage, especially if they are allowed to become stale or contaminated, may increase the occurrence.
- Brush over farrowing house floors that are particularly poor, pitted, and difficult to clean with lime wash containing a phenolic disinfectant.

Scour occurs more frequently in large litters. Split suckling should be implemented.

Colostrum management

It is critical that the piglet receives as much colostrum as possible within the first 12 hours of life. Only during this time period are high quantities of antibody absorbed. Intake is reduced by factors such as poor teat access, poor crate design, and, in particular, the development of agalactia in the sow, which is related with udder oedema. It is critical to determine whether udder oedema is present in a scour outbreak. It occurs more frequently in gilts and second parity sows than in older sows. If E. coli diarrhoea is a problem in younger gilts, it indicates that immunity is low and vaccination should be investigated. Inject the sow twice, two to four weeks apart, with the second injection at least two weeks before farrowing; however, these periods vary according on the vaccination used. Only the gilts should be vaccinated under excellent management conditions.

Treatment

- In severe *E.coli* outbreaks, the sows' diet can be top-dressed with the appropriate antibiotic daily, beginning with admission into the farrowing house and continuing for up to 14 days post-farrowing. This has the potential to reduce bacterial production in sow faeces.
- Examine litters for diarrhoea both at night and in the morning.
- Investigate the disease's history. Is it sporadic, in a single piglet in a litter, or in entire litters?
- In the light of history, either treat the individual pig or treat the entire litter at the first sign of sickness.
- Evaluate the treatment's effectiveness. If there is no improvement after 12 hours, consult your veterinarian and switch to another medication.
- Piglets under 7 days of age should always be treated orally.
- Injections are as beneficial and easier to administer in older pigs.
- Give electrolytes to drinkers. These help to keep the body's electrolytes balanced and avoid dehydration.
- Straw, shredded paper, shavings, or sawdust should be used to cover the pen, creep area, and areas where the pigs defecate.
- Provide a second lamp as an additional source of heat.
- To absorb toxins from the gut, use binding agents such as chalk, kaolin, or activated attapulgite.

Transmissible gastro-enteritis (TGE)

TGE is a serious and extremely contagious piglet disease caused by a corona virus. It is structurally related to but distinct from the corona virus PRCV, which attacks the respiratory system. TGE virus enters the pig via the mouth and multiplies and damages the villi (finger-like structures in the small intestine). This occurs within 24 to 48 hours and is followed by vomiting and severe acute diarrhoea, with a high death rate. When the virus initially enters the herd, mortality in piglets up to 14 days old may be 100%. This diminishes in pigs older than three weeks, although morbidity remains high.

The virus replicates in the intestine and is excreted in vast numbers. Pig faeces are thus the primary source of transmission, either directly via the acquired carrier pig or indirectly via mechanical transmission. The virus is eliminated by sunshine within a few hours, but it can persist outside the pig for extended periods of time in cold or freezing temperatures. It is extremely sensitive to disinfectants, particularly those based on iodine, quaternary ammonia, and peroxygen compounds.

For 2 to 3 weeks, dogs and cats may shed the virus in their faeces. Birds, particularly starlings, can spread the disease, thus managers should ensure that no feed is exposed to attract these birds.

Clinical signs

Weaners and growers

- When the virus is initially introduced into a finishing herd, it causes rapid spread, vomiting, and watery diarrhoea, eventually infecting practically all of the animals.
- The disease goes away on its own after 3 to 5 weeks.
- Typically, mortality is low.
- The primary consequence on the growing pig is dehydration, which resolves in approximately a week.
- Nonetheless, the sickness may delay slaughter by 5-10 days.

Piglets

- The sickness is extremely severe in sucking piglets.
- Acute diarrhoea with water.
- Piglets under 7 days of age died almost entirely within 2 to 3 days due to acute dehydration and electrolyte imbalance.
- Antibiotic treatment has had little effect.
- The moist and muddy hairy appearance of the litter as a result of the profuse diarrhoea is the most noticeable aspect.

Sows

- In acute cases the most prominent feature is the rapidity of spread.
- Vomiting.
- Diarrhoea.
- Adult animals show varying degrees of inappetence.

Diagnosis

In acute disease, the clinical picture is almost diagnostic. There are no other enteric infections that spread so rapidly throughout the pig population. TGE must be diagnosed in a laboratory from the intestine of a fresh dead pig utilising fluorescent antibody tests (FAT's). In addition, the virus is isolated.

PED symptoms are similar to those seen in Transmissible Gastroenteritis (TGE) and Swine Delta Corona Virus (SDCoV) epidemics. While PED and TGE are caused by coronaviruses that are similar, neither virus provides cross immunity.

Causes

- The virus is abundantly excreted in the faeces.
- Pig faeces are thus the primary source of transmission, either directly via the acquired carrier pig or indirectly via mechanical transmission.
- Poor pen hygiene is linked to poor drainage.
- Between pens, poor hygiene procedures
- Environmental pollution from one pen to the next, such as boots, brushes, shovels, clothing, and so on.
- Feeder pipes and bins. This is a high-risk source of enteric disease transmission.
- For 2 to 3 weeks, dogs' faeces may contain the virus.
- Birds, particularly starlings, may spread the disease.
- Feed that has been tainted.
- Continuous use of structures without going all-in, all-out may lead to disease perpetuation.
- Purchase of naive weaners on a regular basis.

Prevention

- When disease is detected, isolate non-infected farrowing houses by utilising separate personnel boots and coveralls. This is especially critical in piglets under 14 days old. The longer the disease is held at bay, the more pigs may be raised and mortality is reduced.
- If feasible, remove sows within three weeks of farrowing from the farm before they become diseased, so they can farrow in an isolated building or outside in arks and avoid sickness.
- Immunity must be developed in dry sows as soon as possible.

- Employ sawdust or shavings in regions where the piglets are scouring. To absorb piglet faeces, paper towels can also be utilised.
- Once the infected period is ended, ensure that the farrowing homes, weaner and finisher accommodation have an all-in and all-out management system.
- Pens should be disinfected between batches using an iodine-based disinfectant or one that is particularly active against viruses.
- This cleaning procedure is critical for preventing the virus from becoming endemic on the farm.
- If your herd has been infected with TGE, inquire why and how. Examine all of your preventative and biosecurity processes.
- Anyone entering your farm should always wear boots and protective attire.
- Disinfectant foot dips should be available at all entries.
- By not exposing starlings and migrating birds to feed, you can keep them away from the farm.
- Borrowing equipment from another pig farm is not permitted.

Place all bins on the unit's exterior and always have your own feeder pipes to your own feed bins. This is a high-risk source of enteric disease transmission.

Treatment

- TGE does not have a specific treatment.
- Individual piglet antibiotic treatment may decrease subsequent infections.
- Make electrolyte-containing water and antibiotics like neomycin readily available. Provide this to the litters twice daily.
- Improve the litter's nursing and habitat by providing extra heat and deep bedding to lower the weights of infection caused by diarrhoea.

Atrophic Rhinitis

Rhinitis is an inflammation of the nose that can be caused by a number of germs and irritants. The delicate structures or turbinate bones in the nose are injured and atrophy or vanish during the infection phase. Progressive atrophic rhinitis is a disorder in which the tissues of the nose permanently atrophy. It is caused by Pasteurella multocidia toxin-producing strains. The carrier pig is nearly always responsible for disease transmission between herds, with the bacterium identified in the respiratory tract and tonsils. Droplet infection between pigs or direct pig-to-pig (nose-to-nose) contact is how it spreads within herds. It can also be spread on equipment, clothing, and other surfaces. Pigs that get infected for the first time can carry the infection for months.

Infection is frequently detected in the second half of the sucking phase or after weaning, and clinical illness can appear as early as three weeks of age. The poison enters the system and harms other tissues such as the liver, kidneys, and lungs, resulting in decreased daily growth and feed efficiency. Although evidence for this is sparse, and there have been no cases of transmission from humans to pigs, the human may carry PMt in the tonsils for a very short amount of time. Experience suggests that carrier pigs are the primary and most likely exclusive source of disease introduction into the herd, while unexplained outbreaks of disease may occur on occasion.

Clinical signs

Sneezing, snuffling, and nasal discharge are the first signs in sucking pigs, but in acute outbreaks where there is insufficient maternal antibodies, the rhinitis can be severe enough to cause nose bleeding. By three to four weeks of age, and beginning with weaning, there is evidence of tear staining and nasal deformity linked with twisting and shortening. Pigs that are severely impacted may have difficulty eating. The daily gain is significantly reduced. Pigs may not reach market weight in severe outbreaks.

Diagnosis

This is determined by clinical indicators. However, do not assume that sneezing in young pigs means they have progressive atrophic rhinitis. Post-mortem inspections of the nose and culture of the organism from nasal swabs easily identify the disease. At slaughter, the snout is sectioned at the level of the second premolar tooth, and the degree of atrophy of the turbinate bones is assessed.

Prevention

- Purchase pigs only from known disease-free sources.
- Inspect snout parts on a regular basis.
- If the herd is infected, do not breed from home-born gilts.
- Sows should be immunised.
- Maintain an aged herd to produce superior colostral immunity.
- Prevent overcrowding, which may allow organisms to collect to the point where they can create a disease outbreak.
- Use all-in-all-out tactics from weaning until slaughter.
- Excessive stocking should be avoided.
- A farrowing room should not have more than ten sows.

- The risk of disease transmission is increased in damp, humid farrowing buildings.
- Establish tight separations between farrowing crates to avoid droplet infection.
- Restrict the number of weaners to no more than 120 per group.
- After weaning, poor ventilation and high humidity are risk factors.

Treatment

- When PAR is diagnosed, all adult stock should be vaccinated twice, 4 to 6 weeks apart, with a toxin-derived vaccine. Vaccination typically provides excellent control.
- Sows should then be vaccinated four to six weeks before the next farrowing.
- Until the clinical epidemic has abated, all weaned piglets should be treated in-feed.
- Antibiotic treatment should be provided to the piglets at the same time, until a good immunity has formed.
- Other antibiotics, such as penicillin, trimethoprim sulphas, tylosin, and enrofloxacin, could be used depending on bacterial sensitivity.
- Starting five to seven days before farrowing and continuing during the farrowing period, the sows' feed could be top-dressed with either OTC or trimethoprim/sulpha (TMS), or the lactation ration could be medicated with trimethoprim/sulpha (TMS) (500g).
- For three weeks after weaning, the creep feed should be treated with OTC or CTC at dose levels of 500-800g/tonne.

Swine Erysipelas

Swine erysipelas is caused by bacteria called Erysipelothrix rhusiopathiae, which is common in nearly all pig farms. Because it is excreted by saliva, faeces, or urine, it is always present in either the pig or the environment. It can survive outside the pig for a few weeks or more in light soils and is found in many other species, including birds and sheep. As a result, it is impossible to eradicate it from a herd.

Infected faeces are most likely the main source of illness. Infection propagation is also aided by contaminated water.

Disease is uncommon in pigs under the age of 8 to 12 weeks due to protection provided by maternal antibodies from the sow via colostrum. Growing pigs, non-vaccinated gilts, and up to fourth parity sows are the most vulnerable.

Although the bacterium can cause the disease on its own, concurrent viral infections, such as porcine reproductive and respiratory syndrome (PRRS) or swine influenza (SI), can induce outbreaks.

The organism enters the body via the tonsils. The pathogen multiplies in the body and enters the bloodstream, resulting in septicaemia. The clinical signs are then determined by the pig's rate of proliferation and level of immunity.

Once a pig gets infected, it develops immunity, which is often linked with moderate or sub-clinical disease.

It can also cause local skin sores in pig. The ability of erysipelas strains to cause disease varies from very minor to extremely severe.

The incubation phase lasts between 24 and 48 hours.

Clinical signs

The onset is abrupt. Typically, the sickness is limited to two or three animals in any given outbreak, though in a non-vaccinated herd, 5 to 10% of animals may be infected at any given time.

Sows

- Death from severe septicaemia or heart failure is frequently the only sign.
- Diamonds are tiny elevated patches of skin caused by a restricted blood supply. These are clearly defined and turn red, then black, due to dead tissue, but there are no abscesses. Most pig recover in 7-10 days.
- Temperatures as high as 108°F fever.
- Clearly unwell.
- Rheumatism is characterised by stiffness or unwillingness to rise.
- Inappetence.
- Infertility.
- Ulceration of the skin.
- The organism affects the joints, causing lameness.
- Abortions with sick sows and dead piglets during acute or subacute illness.
- Mummification and the mortality of piglets in the womb.
- Abortions involving decaying pigs.
- Embryo absorption and delayed returns.
- Litter size varies.

Boars

Boars infected with erysipelas have high temperatures, and sperm might be compromised for the entire five to six week development period.

The significance of erysipelas in reproductive failure

Weaners and growers

- Typically, the condition is less severe and modest.
- Unexpected death.
- Pigs with severe illness are running high temperatures.
- Characteristic skin lesions can also be seen as huge 10 to 50mm elevated diamond-shaped spots all over the body that can become red to black. In the early stages, they may be easier to feel than see, and they usually resolve in 7 to 10 days.
- Despite a high temperature of 107°F, skin sores may emerge, but the pigs may not appear to be ill.
- The organism may settle in the joints, causing chronic arthritis and swellings that can lead to slaughterhouse condemnations.
- Lameness.

Diagnosis

- This is decided by the clinical picture, which includes crucial features such as:
- Inappetence.
- Extremely high temperature.
- Diamond-shaped skin swellings - If the diamond markings are not visible to the naked eye, they can be felt by running your palm over the skin of back, behind back legs, and across flanks.
- A post-mortem examination and isolation of the organism will reveal illness, which is easily grown in the laboratory. The bacterium can cause the disease on its own, but associated virus infections, such as PRRS or influenza, can produce major outbreaks, which should be considered when making a diagnosis.

Causes

- Wet unclean pens, especially if they are extensively contaminated with faeces containing a large number of germs.

- Wet feeding systems, particularly when milk by-products are used, can become important sources of organism proliferation.
- Houses that are constantly occupied with no all-in and all-out processes or disinfection.
- Water systems polluted with the organism.
- Pig movement involves mingling and stress, especially while the sow's maternal antibodies is fading.
- Temperature fluctuations and hot summer weather.
- When pigs dirty their pens during the hot summer months.
- Dietary changes that occur suddenly.
- This is common in straw-based systems.
- Diets high in fungal toxins, especially aflatoxin.
- Heavy parasite burdens or low levels of coccidia allow germs to infiltrate through the damaged intestinal wall.
- Buying non-vaccinated boars or gilts.

Prevention

- If a boar becomes unwell with a fever and skin sores, cure quickly and do not use for mating for at least four weeks.
- Vaccinate all gilts and young boars twice, two to four weeks apart (as directed by the manufacturer), beginning at 14 weeks of age.
- In herds where the challenge is strong, it may be essential to re-vaccinate gilts and boars so that a third dose of vaccination is given two months after the second, usually when breeding animals come on the farm.
- Depending on the incidence and history of disease on the farm, re-vaccinate sows two weeks before farrowing or at weaning.
- Ensure that boars are inoculated every six months.
- If disease breakdowns occur despite immunisation, it is likely that the levels of environmental challenge are considerable. Evaluate breeding pen hygiene and transition to an all-in, all-out housing technique.
- Remember that the organisms can be found in water, faeces, dung, nasal secretions, bedding, and feed during an outbreak.

Treatment

- Penicillin is particularly toxic to the erysipelas bacterium. Acutely unwell animals should be treated for three days with quick acting penicillin.

Alternatively, a long-acting penicillin could be given as a single dosage to cover 48 hours of treatment and then repeated.

- For 10-14 days, medicate the feed with 200g/tonne phenoxymethyl penicillin. This is a very successful way of disease prevention that can be employed in large outbreaks.
- In severe cases, quick-acting penicillin administered twice within the first 24 hours should result in a speedy response. Continue injections three to four days.
- Water medicine with amoxycillin or phenoxy-methyl penicillin should be used when there are a considerable number of sows implicated. The dose will be determined by the purity of the antibiotic powder used.
- Amoxycillin, phenoxymethyl penicillin, and tetracyclines are also effective in drinking water.
- When there are a high number of pigs involved, it may be required to inject all of the pigs in the risk groups.
- Outbreaks encompassing pens or entire pig houses do occur on occasion, particularly during the warmer months.
- If the disease is acute, treatment should begin immediately through the water and be followed by in-feed medication including phenoxymethyl penicillin 200g/tonne or tetracyclines 500g/tonne.
- Finishing pens should be cleansed and disinfected between batches in individual outbreaks. If wet feeding is suspected, the system must be thoroughly cleansed and sterilised.

Anthrax

This acute to chronic condition affects pigs of all ages, but it is more common in grower to adult group. Bacillus anthracis is the causative agent. It is a spore-forming Gram-positive bacillus that generates a protective factor as well as fatal toxins.

Transmission

Infection is usually transmitted through the mouth, but it can also arise as a result of an injection, scratches, or insect bites. The spores are heat resistant and can persist for many years, and contamination of water or soil with them is the most common source of infection. Spores occur when an animal dies or when discharges are exposed to the air, and infected pig flesh or urine, as well as faeces from diseased animals, can spread the disease in a confined space. The disease is most common in ruminants, although it can affect all mammalian species and can be lethal in humans.

Signs

Affected pigs may develop fever to 42 degrees Celsius (107 degrees Fahrenheit), swelling of the neck (pharyngeal form), depression, vomiting, and reluctance to eat, growing trouble in breathing, and death within 24 hours. Some pigs recover, but darkened skin around the swelling site may remain. Fever, digestive trouble, loss of appetite, and the passing of bloody faeces may occur when the infection is localised in the intestine (intestinal form). Death is unusual in this form. Pigs may die if the pathogens induce septicaemia (septicaemic form). Others in the group may experience transitory fever and completely recover, acquire the intestinal form, or have enlarged necks.

Post Mortem lesion

Anthrax is a rare cause of abrupt death, but it should be addressed if fevered animals develop blood-stained faeces or enlargement of the neck consistent with the disease's pharyngeal form. If anthrax is suspected, the corpse should not be opened, and a blood sample from an ear or tissue fluid from the enlarged neck should be collected for laboratory evaluation. There is significant swelling and reddening of the cervical lymph nodes, which are surrounded by gelatinous oedema fluid in the pharyngeal form, as noticed first during post-mortem examination. There may be profuse peritoneal fluid, blackened infarcted patches in the spleen, thickening of the intestinal wall, swelling mediastinal (intestinal) lymph nodes, and adhesion between segments of intestine in the intestinal form. Necrotic (dead) tissue may blanket the intestinal lining. The carcass and its lymph nodes may be reddish, the spleen swollen, and the kidneys petechiated in the septicaemic form (spotted with blood).

Prevention

Anthrax responds to penicillin treatment, and tetracyclines have been used to treat infected animals and remove disease from affected groups by injection, feed, and water. In many countries, governmental veterinarians control the disease since anthrax affects humans and poses a risk to other livestock. While the disease is being handled, the infected farm is usually quarantined. Pigs that are sick are either cured or slaughtered. Because exposure to air permits resistant spores to grow, the bodies of dead afflicted pigs should be cremated or buried unopened. All areas in touch with the carcasses should be cleansed using a spore-killing disinfectant. Slurry from the affected pigs should be disinfected and properly disposed of. The Anthrax Spore Vaccine can protect pigs from the disease in the long run. Because of recent advancements in food safety, meat companies are refusing to take pigs from anthrax-infected herds, and the entire herd may have to be slaughtered, increasing the disease's significance for the pig industry.

Brucellosis

This disease is caused by the bacterium *Brucella suis*. It is an important disease because some strains of it can be transmitted to human where it can cause serious illness. A carrier state persists for long periods of time. It can be spread by venereal infection and the boar is a major source either by direct contact at mating or via artificial insemination. The organism can survive outside the pig for long periods of time particularly at or near freezing temperatures. Pigs can also be infected via the conjunctiva, through the nose or by mouth.

When a female becomes infected, the bacterium multiplies in her blood, resulting in bacteraemia that lasts for 3-6 weeks. During this stage, the bacterium establishes itself in the placenta, causing inflammation and, eventually, abortion. B. suis affects the testicles and accessory reproductive glands and is discharged through the sperm. B. suis, unlike transmissible gastro enteritis (TGE) or foot-and-mouth disease, is not a particularly epizootic infectious bacterium (FMD). It spreads slowly across and within herds, and if you take reasonable care, you should be able to keep it out of your herd. However, it should always be regarded as a dangerous disease.

Clinical signs

Sows

- Bacteraemia
- Infertility.

Boars

- Swollen testicles.
- The infection in the boars' reproductive tract is typically everlasting; the damage that it does is permanent.

Piglets

- Paralysis of hind legs.

Weaners and growers

- Inflamed testicles.
- Lameness.
- Abnormal oestrus.
- Abortions at any time.
- Vulval discharges with pus or sporadically blood.

Causes

- The disease is spread through venereal infection.
- The boar is a significant spreader, either via direct touch during mating or by artificial insemination.
- Through the conjunctiva, the nose, or the mouth.
- Other carriers spread it.
- Deceased piglets, aborted afterbirths, or objects infected with aborted sow vaginal fluids.
- Skin that has been cut or abraded is exposed to infectious materials.
- Suckling sows also excrete the organism in their milk, which infects their piglets.

Prevention

- This is based on identifying and keeping herds free of B. suis infection by acquiring pigs only from disease-free herds.
- Eradication programmes entail finding and eliminating contaminated herds.
- Imported breeding stock was serologically tested.
- Herd blood tests were repeated with positive reactivity removed. This may be beneficial if just a few pigs are sick, but it is unlikely to be useful if a large number of pigs are positive.

Treatment

- Antibiotic treatment is ineffective and should be avoided in most cases.
- Pigs that have been affected should be slaughtered.
- If herd becomes sick, the most dependable management strategy is to cull the herd, clean up the facilities, and replenish with brucella-free pigs. This is also the safest process for pig attendants and the general public, and it is usually the least expensive in the long run.

Greasy pig disease (Exudative epidermitis)

This is caused by the bacterium Staphylococcus hyicus, which infects abraded skin. Toxins produced by Staphylococcus are absorbed into the system and cause liver and kidney damage. Exudative epidermitis, which describes the spilling of fluid from inflamed skin, is another name for the illness. Sow with piglets are usually affected by the disease, but it can be a severe issue in new gilt herds and weaned pigs. It was shown that the bacterium multiplies rapidly in the sow's vagina during the days preceding farrowing. Piglets are frequently infected at or shortly after birth. Only around half of piglets afflicted during suckling survive.

Clinical signs

Small, black, localised spots of infection around the face or on the legs, where the skin has been injured, are typical. The skin on the sides, belly, and between the legs eventually turns brown, affecting the entire body. The skin wrinkles and flakes in huge regions, and it feels greasy. If the sow has given some immunity to the piglet, the image becomes more localised, with little confined lesions 5-10mm in diameter that do not spread. Disease may emerge two to three days after weaning in weaned pigs, beginning with a minor browning of the skin and progressing to a dark greasy texture, and in severe cases, the skin turns black. Toxins produced by staphylococci organisms generally cause death in such circumstances. Up to 15% of the population may be involved in nurseries.

Sows

Unusual but localised lesions may be seen mainly behind the face and eyes.

Piglets

- Piglets with severe illnesses will die.
- On the flanks and behind the ears, there are lesions. Lesions generally start as tiny, dark, localised areas of infection on the face or legs.
- Eventually, the skin on the sides, belly, and between the legs turns brown, affecting the entire body.
- The skin is wrinkled and flaky in large areas, and it feels oily.
- Necrosis causes the skin to turn black and the piglets to perish in severe cases.
- If the sow has given the piglet some immunity, the picture becomes more localised, with small restricted lesions 5-10mm in diameter that do not spread.

Weaners and growers

- Generally, three days after weaning, localised, black areas of infection or dermatitis appear around the face or on the legs where the skin has been wounded. Ulcers could form.
- Eventually, the skin on the sides, belly, and between the legs turns brown, affecting the entire body.

- In large areas, the skin wrinkles and peels.
- It darkens and becomes oily, and in severe cases, it turns black.
- Toxins released by staphylococci species usually result in mortality in such situations.
- Nurseries may employ up to 15% of the population.
- Dehydration is fairly common.

Diagnosis

This is based on the typical skin lesions. It is critical to culture the organism and perform an antibiotic sensitivity test during an outbreak. A moist wet region should be located, the covering scab should be removed, and a swab should be rubbed well into the affected area. This should be returned to the laboratory as quickly as possible, preferably within 24 hours, in a transport medium.

Causes

- The sharp eye teeth cut the skin around the mouth during a teat competition.
- It may also be triggered by sucking abrasions on the knees.
- Abrasions from bad concrete surfaces or metal floors, as well as side panels.
- Faulty iron injection techniques, as well as tail and tooth removal.
- Fighting and skin damage occur during weaning.
- Mange causes skin injury.
- Metal feeding troughs can cause face injuries, leading to illness.
- Abnormal behaviour includes tail biting, ear biting, navel sucking, and flank biting.
- At birth, the teeth were poorly trimmed.

Prevention

- Examine the pigs to see where abrasions are occurring. These could be caused by fresh concrete surfaces or harsh metal flooring, for example.
- If concrete surfaces are in poor condition, brush them down after cleaning with hydrated lime containing a phenol disinfectant.
- Examine the methods for removing tails and teeth. Teeth with jagged edges can cause gum injury and infection around the cheeks, especially when piglets battle for teat access and during mixing after weaning.

- One reservoir of infection is the udder skin. This should be sprayed with an iodine-based skin antiseptic three days before and after farrowing (cow teat dip is ideal).
- Clean the flooring thoroughly between farrowings.
- Ensure that needles used for iron injections are changed between litters on a regular basis.
- If the herd has mange, treat the sow before she enters the farrowing house.
- Extreme humidity and damp pens might encourage the bacteria to multiply.
- Metal floors and side panels, particularly braided metal flooring, can inflict serious abrasions on the feet and legs. The earliest signs of greasy pig will appear in these places in such circumstances. Metal feeding troughs can cause facial injuries, which can lead to sickness.
- Check the humidity of the weaning environment. High levels exceeding 70% and high temperatures create an excellent habitat for bacteria to multiply on the skin.
- Adopt an all-in, all-out approach to weaning accommodations.

Treatment

- Determine antibiotic sensitivity in infected piglets and inject them daily for five days, or on alternate days, with a long-acting antibiotic to which the organism is sensitive.
- Amoxycillin, OTC, ceftiofur, cephalexin, gentamycin, lincomycin, or penicillin are examples of antibiotics.
- Antibiotics used topically may also be beneficial. Novobiocin, an antibiotic used to treat mastitis in dairy cows, can be combined with mineral oil and sprayed into the skin or dipped into a solution.
- Piglets become dehydrated and should be given electrolytes orally.
- Ascertain that the herd is free of mange. Mange mites cause skin injury and allow Staphylococcus hyicus to enter.
- Long-acting injections can be administered two to three days before the first symptoms occur as a preventative measure. If indicated, use either long-acting amoxycillin or oxytetracyclin.
- In severe outbreaks, an autogenous vaccine made from the organism can be developed and given into sows twice, four and two weeks before farrowing, to boost immunity in the colostrum. This has worked well on several farms where illness has arisen in both sucking and weaning piglets.

- If the problem occurs in gilt litters, cross suckling these piglets at birth with older sows for four or five hours can be beneficial.

Leptospirosis

Leptospira are spiral-shaped bacteria that live in the majority of mammalian hosts. Once introduced into a herd, the pigs become permanent carriers, developing kidney disease and excreting the organism in their urine on occasion. Leptospira can become localised in the uterus during pregnancy, resulting in abortions or an increase in stillborn piglets. Leptospira can also be found in sow fallopian tubes and boar reproductive organs, and it is transmitted through sperm. This could be an important pathway for infection maintenance in the herd and the cause of sow infertility. Disease is rare in sucking pigs.

The symptoms of leptospirosis can be misguided for other causes of infertility including:

- Chronic porcine reproductive and respiratory syndrome (PRRS).
- Endometritis.
- Non-infectious causes.
- Summer infertility.
- Management failures.

Clinical signs

Piglets

- Unusual.
- Inappetence.
- Jaundice.
- Blood in urine.

Sows

- Inappetence.
- Fever.
- Depression may be observed.
- Abortions.
- Stillbirths.
- Increase in poor, non-viable pigs.

Weaners and growers

- Acute jaundice.
- Haemorrhage.
- Rapid death.
- Pale pigs.

Diagnosis

Leptospirosis can be difficult to diagnose because pigs are frequently infected yet exhibit no clinical signs. The primary method of diagnosis is to assess antibody levels in a sample of breeding females and isolate the organism from diseased tissues. Leptospirosis must be distinguished from other causes of infertility.

Causes

Infected gilts and boars are introduced.

AI can potentially contaminate a herd if no antibiotics are used in the sperm.

Infection spread by other animals; rats, mice, and dogs can serve as reservoirs of infection. The herd is exposed to indirect sources of contamination, such as contaminated water and poor floor surfaces, which allow urine to pool. Unless extreme precautions are taken, most herds will be exposed at some point. Infection occurs through the mouth, via the mucous membranes. The majority of leptospira is discovered in urine and lives in the kidney. Venereal infection is extremely prevalent.

Prevention

- Routine immunisation of breeding stock is prevalent in nations where the organism is enzootic, but less so in border and free zones. The vaccination, like all bacterial vaccines (bacterins), does not confer complete immunity but usually increases resistance enough to prevent clinical symptoms. The utilised vaccines are inactivated and contain an adjuvant. Vaccines containing five or six different strains of leptospira are available in several countries.
- Alternatively, where immunisations are unavailable, antimicrobial therapy must be used.
- When leptospira become active and present in the herd, sanitation, frequent urine removal, and effective management become critical ways of control.

- The most effective technique of control is to offer two wallows per paddock and utilise an electric fence to allow each to alternately dry out and relax.
- Poor concrete surfaces that collect urine and water are suitable sources for maintaining high levels of infection in indoor dwellings.
- Ensure that concrete surfaces are well-drained, especially in defecating areas and boar pens.
- If the sow is only exposed to a small number of germs, infection will most likely occur with little illness.
- Keep rodents in check.
- Contamination from pig vehicles is a low risk in comparison to other illnesses.
- Slurry should be removed on a regular basis.
- In cases when there is a history of recurrent infertility, in-feed medicine can be administered immediately before the expected onset of disease.
- If streptomycin is available, inject 25mg/kg into sows at weaning time. This medicine should be given to boars every six weeks. Semi-synthetic penicillins could also be employed.
- After service, inject an antibiotic into the anterior vagina. This is the same technique as described under vaginal discharges, and it entails inserting an AI catheter and injecting antibiotics into the anterior vagina 6-18 hours after the last mating. It is possible to utilise ampicillin, amoxycillin, or penicillin/dihydrostreptomycin.

Treatment

Tetracyclines, either oxytetracycline or chlortetracycline, at 800g/tonne, should be added to the feed. Feed for three weeks, then repeat the process six weeks later, and so on for four treatment periods.

Mastitis, Metritis, Agalactia (MMA)

- Mastitis, metritis, and agalactia (MMA) is a complicated condition seen in sows shortly after farrowing. A bacterial infection of the mammary glands and urogenital tract causes it. MMA causes higher piglet mortality and lower weaning weights.
- **Mastitis** An udder bacterial infection. Often, only one or two glands are damaged.
- **Metritis** A uterine infection characterised by vulval discharges

- **Agalactia** Sow milk production is reduced or lost entirely. It is frequently not identified until the nursing litter exhibits signs of hunger and weight loss.

Clinical signs

Clinical indicators include constipation, fever, and anorexia, in addition to mastitis, metritis, and agalactia. Inappetence is frequently the initial symptom, followed by restlessness during suckling and a loss of condition in the litter. Few MMA cases exhibit all of the symptoms at the same time, and the symptoms are usually farm-specific. In some circumstances, limited milk supply and piglet daily liveweight gain may be the only signs of a problem.

Diagnosis

Clinical symptoms, particularly inappetence un the sow and a decrease in litter condition, are used to make the diagnosis. By passing a hand under both lines of glands, the udder can be palpated on both sides; afflicted glands will feel firm and heated. Mastitis can be diagnosed by analysing the milk; collection will necessitate an oxytocin injection to encourage milk let down.

The litter should also be inspected because diarrhoea, septicaemia, or hypothermia can cause decreased milk intake and an oversupply of milk in the udder, which can cause drying off.

Control and Prevention

- The most effective MMA prevention measure is cleanliness.
- To avoid bacterial problems, the farrowing pen and sow must be kept clean and dry at this time. A thorough cleaning and disinfection technique is required.
- Sows who exercise more before farrowing and in the early stages of nursing may have a lower risk of developing MMA.
- Prevent slick floors, which are a primary cause of decreased activity in lactating sows.
- Sows that are overweight are more vulnerable to MMA, as are sows that have been overfed prior to farrowing.
- Ensure sows have constant access to water; lactating sows require 15 to 30 litres per day.

Treatment

- A good drainage system can keep sows clean and dry.

- Always seek the counsel of your veterinarian while dealing with MMA.
- Antibiotics and medications to minimise inflammation are commonly used in treatment, as is the injection of chemicals to encourage milk production.
- Small doses of oxytocin can aid, but they should not be required if piglets are suckling frequently; oxytocin, if taken early on, may lessen the need for veterinary intervention.
- Treatment should begin as soon as MMA is identified or if the sow's body temperature increases above 39.4°C 12 to 18 hours after farrowing.
- The sow should be urged to drink by urging her to rise on a frequent basis.

Some sows recover without treatment, but by that time, the litter will have suffered.

- Once a problem litter is recognised, efforts should be taken to prevent dehydration, provide an alternative source of energy, and increase milk supply.
- Small piglets may need to be moved soon to another sow with a high milk production rate.
- Strict hygiene is required to reduce the risk of metritis.
- Consult your veterinarian about if it is necessary to administer antibiotics after interfering.
- Keep the sows back clean and dry, and ensure there are no leaking drinkers.

Roundworm Infection (Ascariasis)

Ascariasis is a swine infection caused by the roundworm Ascaris suum, which can cause pneumonia, hepatitis, and malnutrition.

Clinical signs

Unthriftiness, failure to gain weight, rough hair coat, pendulous abdomen, recurrent paroxysmal coughing, and, on rare occasions, abdominal expiratory dyspnea are symptoms in young, growing pigs. Severe, sometimes deadly, pulmonary disease can occur 7-14 days after naive pigs are placed in substantially contaminated facilities with ascarid eggs. Afebrile pigs "thump," are emaciated, and are frequently misdiagnosed as having bacterial or viral pneumonia. Other adverse consequences in extensively exposed gilts include delayed estrus, a low conception rate, pneumonia, and death.

Lesions

Small haemorrhages appear on and across the lungs 5-14 days following ingestion of infective eggs. Smaller airways are obstructed by larvae and inflammatory exudate (verminous pneumonia). Secondary suppurative bronchopneumonia is common. The pneumonia may be accompanied by emphysema, which prevents the lungs from collapsing. Scarring in the liver begins 7-14 days after exposure as scattered grey to white "milk spots" (0.2-1 cm) visible under the liver capsule, which later grow, consolidate, and resolve. In severe infections, diffuse fibrosis can damage the entire liver, condemning it to slaughter. Minor scarring can be restored in 30 to 60 days, casting doubt on the diagnostic reliability of detecting the absence of liver abnormalities at slaughter.

Control

To make timely and cost-effective deworming decisions, a thorough understanding of the life cycle of ascarids and the infestation status of a herd or group of pigs is essential.

Ascariasis prevention is considerably superior to treatment, however it may be difficult to implement on many manufacturing sites. Swine raised in confinement with an effective ascariasis management programme have few ascarids. Deworming the sows during gestation; washing the sows to remove parasite eggs prior to putting them in sanitised farrowing crates; early weaning of two to four week old pigs; and using all in/all out production systems with thorough cleaning between groups are some of the measures that confinement operators implement.

Pigs raised in hygienic confinement systems are frequently clear of ascarid infection until they are placed in contaminated facilities. As a result of ingesting countless eggs from the environment, these pigs may get acute pneumonia. In this circumstance, feeding a continuous dewormer for the first 30 days is a control alternative. To avoid further egg contamination, pigs in such settings should be dewormed at no more than eight-week intervals.

Deworming sows before shifting them to clean pasture is a useful technique in enterprises that use pasture or open lot housing. Pasture rotation reduces swine exposure to worm eggs significantly, especially if the ground is tilled while not pastured. Deworming treatments must be tailored to the needs of each production location.

Anthelmintics should be chosen based on the full range of nematode species found on the farm, including ascarids. A monitoring system must be established and implemented. The parasite problem can alter as a result of the introduction of new parasites, facility changes, or climatic changes, all of which can affect the amount and type of parasites.

Coccidiosis

Coccidiosis is caused by coccidia, which are microscopic parasites that dwell and proliferate inside host cells, primarily in the intestine. Eimeria, Isospora, and Cryptosporidia are the three types. Disease is common and pervasive in sucking piglets and, on rare occasions, in pigs as young as 15 weeks. The predominant clinical symptom is diarrhoea.

Clinical signs

- Coccidiosis induces diarrhoea in piglets due to minor intestinal wall injury. As a result, secondary bacterial infections develop.
- Dehydration is fairly common.
- The consistency and colour of the faeces vary depending on the severity of the condition, ranging from yellow to grey green or scarlet.
- Despite the fact that death from coccidiosis is relatively rare, secondary infection by bacteria and viruses can result in considerable mortality.
- Sickness has been found in young boars and gilts confined in permanently occupied cages and fed on the floor on occasion.

Diagnosis

Coccidiosis should be suspected if there is diarrhoea in sucking piglets aged 7-21 days that does not react well to medications. In some outbreaks, however, diagnosis is challenging because finding oocysts in the faeces of infected pigs might be difficult. In some outbreaks, however, post-mortem exams reveal unambiguous indications. The oocysts do not pass out into the faeces until roughly 3-4 days after the pig has recovered from diarrhoea. Faeces samples for laboratory analysis should be collected from semi-recovered pigs rather than scour pigs.

Prevention

- Once the oocysts have established themselves in a habitat, the sow becomes secondary. Other than flies, dried faeces, dust, and feces-contaminated surfaces, oocysts pollute the environment. Insect control and hygiene are critical.
- Daily removal of sow and piglet faeces.
- Improve farrowing house hygiene, particularly farrowing pen flooring, and prevent faeces from moving from one pen to another.
- Ensure that slurry tubes are fully empty between farrowings as much as feasible.

- Wash and disinfect the farrowing houses thoroughly with OO-CIDE (Antec) or other anti-oocyst chemicals.
- If the farrowing crate floor surfaces are concrete and pitted, brush them with lime wash and allow them to dry before the next sow arrives.
- Keep the pens as dry as possible, especially the parts of the floor where the piglets defecate. Covering wet areas with shavings and removing them everyday is an excellent strategy.
- If creep is fed on the floor, it should be stopped until the piglets are at least 21 days old.
- Fly control.
- Wallows can be a great source of infection, especially during lactation. Increase the quantity of shade and make sprays available.
- Site wallows far from the food supply.

Treatment

- This must be taken immediately prior to the invasion of the intestinal wall for it to be effective. The damage has been done once clinical indications arise.
- Medicate the sow feed using 1kg/tonne amprolium premix, 100g/tonne monensin sodium, or 100g/tonne sulphadimidine. Feed the sow from the time she enters the farrowing house until the end of lactation.
- At six days of age, inject each litter with a long-acting suphonamide.
- Medicate small amounts of milk powder with a coccidiostat such as amprolium or salinomycin and administer to piglets starting at three days of age, top dressed on creep feed.
- Toltrazuril at a dose of 6.25mg/kg is successful in managing illness in one or two doses. It is made by combining 250ml of glycerol, 125ml of water, and 125ml of Baycox. A 2ml dose can be administered once at 4, 5, or 6 days of age, depending on the response, and then repeated at ten days of age.

Endoparasites (internal parasites)

The enormous white worms ascarids (Ascaris suum), red stomach worms (Hyostrongylus rubidus), and whip worms are the most important parasites in the sow. To reproduce and thrive, all of these parasites must consume resources from the host. They can be detected in the gastrointestinal system, he kidneys, the liver, the lungs, or the bloodstream.

The sow becomes a possible source of infection for the piglets. In the piglet, the threadworm (Strongyloides ransomi) is significant.

Internal parasites are uncommon in weaned, growing, and finishing pigs unless they are housed in constantly inhabited straw-based or bare concrete pens, where ascarids may become a concern.

There are four groups of endoparasitic worms: nematodes (roundworms); thorny-headed worms; tapeworms and protozoa:

Clinical signs

Sows

- Coughing.
- Loss of body condition.
- Hairy pigs.
- Vomiting.
- Blood in faeces.
- Anaemia.
- Diarrhoea
- Piglets
- Coughing.
- Stiffness.
- Pain.
- Vomiting.
- Bloody diarrhoea.
- Some morality.

Weaners and growers

- Diarrhoea
- poor growth and sloppy faeces
- Coughing.
- Blood infaeces.
- Pneumonia and heavy breathing.
- Pale pigs.

Diagnosis

This is based on symptoms and recognition of the parasites.

Laboratory testing of faeces for worm eggs.

Causes

- Management systems that permit frequent access to faeces.
- Allowing faeces to remain in shed for longer than 3 - 4 days
- Eggs thrive in moist, humid environments.
- There will be no all-in, all-out management.
- Failure to carry out routine treatments as prescribed.
- Constantly used pens raise the danger of infection.
- Muddy, wet floors.
- Carrier Pigs.

Prevention

Parasite control necessitates a grasp of their life cycle. Procedures that, in conjunction with anthelmintics, disrupt the cycle and so prevent re-infection can then be implemented.

Treatment

Controlled application of anthelmintics.

Agent	Common Name	Piperazine	Pyrantel	Avermectins	Levamisole	Dichlorvos	Fenbendazole
Stephanurus dentatus	Kidneyworm	-	-	+	+	-	+
Haematopinus suis	Lice	-	-	+	-	-	-
Metastrongylus spp.	Lungworm	-	-	+	+	-	+
Sarcoptes scabiei	Mange mite	-	-	+	-	-	-
Oesophagostomum spp.	Nodular worm	+	+	+	+	+	+
Ascaris suum	Roundworm	+	+	+	+	+	+
Macracanthorhynchus hirudinaceus	Thorny-headed worm	-	-	-	-	-	-
Strongyloides ransomi	Threadworm	-	-	+	+	-	-
Trichuris suis	Whipworm	-	-	-	+	+	+

Ectoparasites

Ectoparasites are parasites that live outside the body, and their relevance varies widely across locations due to variations in climate and pig-raising system types. These parasites feed and multiply on the host animal at the expense of the pig, and they are especially harmful to young and growing pigs. The additional stress caused by a parasite infestation might result in poor weight growth, requiring more feed per kilogramme of gain than an uninfected pig. External parasites in pigs cause a variety of clinical indications such as rubbing, scratching, and skin sores. Some parasites can have major economic consequences since they affect growth rate, feed efficiency, and carcass value at slaughter.

Pig mange mite

The mange mite is the most common external parasite of pigs worldwide. The sarcoptes mite is a small, greyish-white, circular parasite that is only visible to the human eye when put against a dark background.

Acute disease

Ear shaking and intense rubbing of the skin against the sides of the pen are common symptoms. Approximately three to eight weeks after the first infection, the skin becomes sensitised to the mite protein, and a severe allergy with extremely minute red spots covering the entire skin may develop in susceptible individuals. Severe rubbing and bleeding may develop as a result of the intense irritation.

Chronic disease

Following the acute phase, thick encrustations containing mites form on the ear, the sides of the neck, the elbows, the front sections of the hocks, and the top of the neck.

Diagnosis

The presence of the mite in the herd confirms the diagnosis of sarcoptic mange. The ideal way is to use a torch to inspect the inside surface of animals' ears for encrusted lesions. Encrusted lesions can be scraped off using an object, such as a teaspoon, and placed on a black sheet of paper for 10 minutes. After 10 minutes, turn the paper upside down to remove the scabs; any mites on the paper will stick to it and can be seen with the naked eye with a magnifying glass.

Maintenance of mange-free pig farm

The mite dies quickly in the environment, often lasting up to five days in most agricultural environments but up to four weeks in damp, sheltered conditions. Mites are susceptible to drying, and if exposed to direct sunlight or dry conditions, they will die within 24 to 48 hours. This is a crucial aspect of control. Mange is one of the easiest illnesses to keep out of a herd when it is clear of it because it can only be introduced by carrier pigs. However, once established, it typically becomes endemic unless control measures are implemented. Exposure to situations where the mites are still living can result in infection in as little as 24 hours in immature pigs.

The establishment and maintenance of mange-free herds is expedited by three important facts:

- Mite-free piglets are born;
- Mites are very host-specific and do not live long away from their host; and
- Modern treatments are highly effective.

Control

Mange control entails identifying animals with chronic mange so that they can undergo systematic and consistent treatment to safeguard the herd's younger animals. All control programmes must concentrate on the breeding herd. All animals with significant hyperkeratotic lesions in the ears and throughout the body should be culled, and the remaining sows should be treated concurrently or in segregated groups prior to farrowing.

Contaminated bedding should be removed and shed sprayed with insecticide.

Treat all pigs on a regular basis to avoid a buildup of numbers.

- Boars should be treated every three months.
- Always give animals two treatments, 10 to 15 days apart.
- After diseased pigs have been removed from the pens, clean, disinfect, and dry the pens before spraying with a suitable pesticide.

Mange-free herds can be established through depopulation and repopulation from mange-free animals, segregated upbringing of treated pigs, or eradication using 'avermectin' type products and other registered products.

Implementing bio-security measures, particularly isolating and treating incoming stock and procuring stock from a small number of herds, is usually sufficient to prevent parasite reintroduction.

Sarcoptic Mange

Mange is a parasitic skin disease caused by either Sarcoptes scabiei or Demodex phylloides mites. Sarcoptic mange (also known as scabies) is by far the most prevalent and serious because it is irritating and uncomfortable for the pig, forcing it to rub and destroy the skin, making it ugly. It has a considerable impact on growth rate and feed efficiency.

The mite spreads from pig to pig directly through skin contact or contact with freshly contaminated surfaces. Because pig is always in direct skin contact with breeding females and is a chronic carrier, the boar aids in the spread of infection in the herd. Pigs housed in groups have a greater chance of spreading. Under most agricultural conditions, the mite dies out swiftly away from the pig in less than five days. This is a crucial aspect of control. If a herd is mange-free, it is one of the simplest diseases to keep at bay because it can only be introduced by carrier pigs. However, once introduced, it becomes persistently endemic unless control measures are implemented.

Field observations suggest that after eradication, sows are less restless, resulting in lower piglet mortality and higher weaning weights. The most significant benefits, however, are an increase in feed efficiency of up to 0.1 and an increase in daily liveweight gain of 4 to 10% depending on severity.

Clinical signs

Piglets

- Skin irritation after 7 days.

Sows

Weaners and growers

- Its presence has an impact on food conversion and daily gain, especially if the infection is significant.
- Tiny red pimples appear all over the skin.
- Itching and rubbing/scratching.
- Chronic disorder characterised by thick asbestos-like scabs primarily on the ears, typically with minor bleeding and constant rubbing.
- Poor growth.
- Ear shaking.

Causes

- The mite spreads from pig to pig by close skin contact or contact with recently contaminated surfaces.

- The boar contributes to the spread of infection in the herd because boar is always in direct physical contact with breeding females and is a chronic carrier.
- Pigs housed in groups are more likely to spread.
- Pigs that have lately been purchased.
- When sows are housed in groups, disease spreads more easily.
- Pens were always housed.

Prevention

Mange is a costly disease not just because of the economic consequences for the pig, but also because of the expenditures and necessity for frequent treatment.

Treatment

Spraying, putting an oily liquid containing phosmet 20% to the rear of the pig (the treatment is absorbed via the skin), or in-feed medication or injection can all be used to control the disease. The ultimate goal of any management effort, however, must be to remove the parasite.

Some Drugs Used in the treatment of Mange (for specific uses and withdrawal periods see the relevant manufacturers data sheets)

Trade Name/salt	Method of Application	Comments
Amitraj 0.1%	Spray, Pour on	3 times 10 days apart
Benzyl benzoate	Topical Application	Chronic lesion
Diazin on 0.05%	Spray	3 times 10 days apart
Doramectin	Injection	Repeat in 14 days, 49 days withdrawl
Ivermectin	Feed Injection	Repeat in 14 days
Lindane 0.06%	Spray	Repeat in 14 days, 60 days withdrawl
Malathion 0.5%	Spray	Repeat in 14 days
Phosmet 20%	Pour on	Repeat in 14 days
Toxaphene 0.5%	Spray	Repeat in 14 days

Demodectic Mange

In pigs, this mite is thought to be insignificant. It is found in hair follicles. Treatment is ineffective; however the mite is sensitive to acaricides used to cure sarcoptic mange. Animals who are severely afflicted should be removed from the herd.

Louse Infestation (Pediculosis)

Infestation is widespread in areas with inadequate husbandry and management. The lice only survive on swine, yet they may infest individuals who work with swine. Swine of all ages are vulnerable to infestation. The infestation is worse in the winter, but it is there all year. The parasitism is most likely present everywhere swine are farmed.

Haematopinus suis is one of the largest lice species, measuring up to 6 mm in length. Haematopinus suis is a sucking louse that feeds on blood from the host via its penetrating mouth parts. The louse lives on the host its entire life. It can only survive for a few days without the host. The female louse lives for around 23-30 days, lays three to four eggs every day, and attaches them to the base of hair shafts. Eggs are 1-2 mm long and range in hue from light cream to grey. They hatch between 12 and 20 days.

Hog lice, like the majority of lice, are host specific. They typically spread among pigs when they are in close proximity, such as when they gather together for warmth, shade, or comfort. Lice can also spread to pigs that are transferred into quarters that have recently been abandoned by lousy animals. Infested animals introduced into a clean herd frequently introduce lice.

Because lice prefer to feed on thin-skinned areas, they have specific favoured spots on a pig. The neck, jowl, flank, inside side of the thighs, and ears are also popular locations. Because it is difficult to properly moisten the inside surface of the ear, lice are protected from parasiticides.

When lice enter the skin to feed on blood, they annoy swine. Dermatitis develops, causing rubbing, scratching, and hair loss. Most pigs do not suffer from blood loss, but it can cause severe anaemia in nursing piglets and make them more prone to other diseases. Pigs that have been parasitized are agitated. They could lose weight and eat less efficiently.

Lice are known vectors of swine pox, African swine disease, and eperythro-zoonosis. Other infectious agents may also be transmitted, it appears.

Clinical signs

Pediculosis is characterised by persistent rubbing and itching, patchy baldness, and pallor. Because sarcoptic mange exhibits similar symptoms, it must be distinguished. Pediculosis and sarcoptic mange are frequently found together. Hog lots and facilities with numerous rubbing areas may also indicate the presence of lice or mange.

Diagnosis

A rough, drab hair coat is common in lesions, as is patchy alopecia. An extensive examination reveals lice and ova adhering to the hair. Examining the inside of the ears frequently reveals lice, and it is also a good location to look for sarcoptic mange sores.

Picking up a few little and growing pigs, turning them over, and inspecting their undersides is a useful practise. Lice, as well as lesions from a variety of other disorders, are frequently seen on the posterior belly or the inside surface of the legs.

The punctate cutaneous lesions induced by feeding lice are noticeable at slaughter and hair removal, especially in white-skinned hogs.

Treatment and control

Before being brought into a herd, animals should always be treated with a parasiticide, ideally twice at two-week intervals. There are numerous effective parasiticides available today. A second treatment kills lice that hatch from eggs 12-20 days after the first treatment.

Other than lice, several parasiticides are used to control external parasites (flies, mites and ticks). Injectable avermectins have proven to be particularly effective in eliminating lice and mange, and strategies for eradicating both have been developed.

Control and eradication procedures for sarcoptic mange also apply to lice. These include paying specific attention to the ears, treating the boars, several treatments of sows before to farrowing, separating clean and untreated animals if the entire herd is not treated at the same time, and treating all introduced animals.

Ticks/ Flies/ Mosquitoes

Ticks

Ticks infest many species of mammals and birds and are not host-specific.

Ticks are easily seen with the naked eye, and their size and appearance vary depending on whether or not they have recently fed. They can be found anywhere on the body, although they are more commonly found on the softer skin of the ears, neck, and flanks.

Tick treatment and control in pigs is rarely necessary. If only a few ticks are present, they can be manually removed with a tick removal instrument and the pigs confined away from the contaminated area. Treatments for lice are usually effective.

Flies

Some flies disturb animals with their violent bites, while others serve as a vector for infectious disease transmission.

They can irritate pigs by biting (depending on the fly species) and become major carriers of disease-causing organisms such as pathogenic strains of E. coli, B. hyodysenteriae, salmonella, streptococci, and rotavirus.

Fly populations can exacerbate major outbreaks of greasy pig disease and coccidiosis, and when sows have mastitis, flies are attracted to the udder and skin surfaces in large numbers, and they can be responsible for exacerbating severe outbreaks.

Fly control in all piggeries is must during the summer months to prevent flies from breeding and to eliminate adult flies. Fly breeding can be avoided by regularly removing dung and use baited fly traps and pesticides.

Mosquitoes

Mosquitoes bite producing pain at best and severe irritation at worst. Lesions in the form of elevated oedematous weals on the legs and abdomen can arise on several or all of the piglets. Mosquitoes play a vital role in the transmission of the Japanese encephalitis virus and serve as mechanical vectors for the spread of Eperythrozoon suis. Mosquito bites can upset nursing sows, leading to piglet mortality.

To reduce the population of mosquitos, numerous control strategies can be applied. When there is a disease outbreak, fogging may be used to destroy the infected adult mosquito population, and local governments may employ larvicides to prevent human infection. Wherever possible, mosquito breeding grounds should be discovered and larvae eliminated by draining water reservoirs or coating the surface with environmentally safe oil.

Anaemia

Anaemia is a disorder characterised by a decrease in the quantity of red blood cells, the amount of haemoglobin they contain, or the volume of the red cells themselves.

It might manifest itself in one of three ways:

Blood loss due to haemorrhage. Examples include gastrointestinal ulcers, vulva damage, and a ruptured liver.

Inadequate haemoglobin levels related to nutritional deficiencies, particularly iron and copper.

Red cell count has decreased. These are made in the bone marrow, and any sickness, infection, or toxic state that affects it can cause anaemia.

Anaemia is also frequently seen as a secondary clinical symptom of other disorders, such as actinobacillus pleuropneumonia or glässers disease.

Clinical signs

Piglets

Piglets become pale and growth is occasionally delayed. The skin's colour may appear slightly yellow or jaundiced. In extreme cases, breathing is fast, especially during exertion, and there may be a proclivity to scour.

All pigs

- Pale skin tone.
- Rapid breathing.
- Jaundiced on occasion
- Pale mucous membranes of the eyes.
- Sloppy diarrhoea, scour.
- Haemorrhage symptoms.
- Weakness.
- There may be an increase in stillbirths.
- Haemorrhage can be visible on the outside or occur through bleeding into the tissues or the intestines.

Diagnosis

Anaemia can be diagnosed clinically and by studying a blood sample. This is done to determine the red cell volume and haemoglobin levels. A stained blood smear will also confirm the shape and size of the red cells, as well as the presence of germs. The various anaemias are caused by certain cell types. Piglets may develop anaemia as a result of iron dextran toxicity combined with vitamin E insufficiency.

Causes

- Gastric ulcers
- Haematoma
- Internal bleeding

- Loss of blood
- Porcine enteropathy
- Prolapse of the rectum
- Torsion of the stomach and intestines
- Faulty nutrition.
- Lack of iron or copper.
- Warfarin poisoning.

Prevention

Piglets

The simplest technique is to give the piglet a 1 or 2ml injection of 150-200 mg iron dextran.

Iron is best provided between the ages of 3 and 5 days, rather than at birth.

The injection sites are either the muscles of the hind leg or the neck. Use a needle with a gauge of 21 (5/8 inch).

Iron can also be provided orally, but this method takes time and requires the pig to be treated twice or three times at 7, 10, and 15 days of age.

Ad lib oral pastes have been tried, however intake within every litter is varied, and a few piglets remain anaemic.

All pigs

Regular deworming programmes and/or parasite testing of faeces samples every 3 to 6 months, as well as monitoring iron levels in diet, should be implemented.

Treatment

- The intestine can only absorb a limited amount of iron every day, which may not be enough to immediately correct anaemia. Nonetheless, the iron and copper levels in the feed should be monitored. It is also beneficial to administer a 300-500mg injection of iron dextran depending on the age of the pig.
- The cause will determine the specific treatment and prevention.
- Electrolytes can be given via injection or by mouth in extreme situations.

Porcine Stress Syndrome (PSS)

This term refers to a set of disorders caused by an autosomal recessive gene. Acute stress and rapid death (malignant hypothermia), pale soft exudative muscle (PSE), dark firm dry meat, and back muscular necrosis are all part of it. Pigs with a lot of muscle are more likely to have the gene.

Clinical signs

Sows

- The onset is sudden.
- Muscle tremors are noticeable.
- Twitching of the mouth.
- Rapid breathing.
- The skin turns red and blotchy.
- Death normally takes about 15-20 minutes.
- A notable trait is the rapid onset of rigour mortis.
- Temperature rise of more than 106 degrees F.

Weaners and growers

- The onset is abrupt, accompanied by muscle tremors.
- Twitching of the mouth.
- Rapid breathing.
- The skin turns red
- Death normally takes about 15-20 minutes.
- Back muscular necrosis is a less severe variant of PSS.
- While the gene results in a slimmer carcass, growth rates are slower and the incidence of premature mortality rises.

Prevention

- Take the gene out of the population.
- If the gene is to be employed to improve carcase quality, use a homozygous or heterozygous male on stress gene free females.
- Keep your herd gene-free.

Treatment

- This is usually ineffectual, but the following steps should be taken:
- To control temperature spikes, spray the pig with cold water.
- In two separate intramuscular injections, administer 50-100ml of calcium gluconate. Seek veterinary assistance.
- Use stresnil to sedate the pig.
- Avoid moving or causing excessive muscle activation.
- Give a 2iu/kg injection of vitamin E.

Some other pig diseases

Listeriosis

The bacterium Listeria monocytogenes causes this, and it can colonise the tonsils and be passed out in faeces. Listeria is common in nature and is frequently detected in cheese and silage. Infection occurs as a result of exposure, but illness is uncommon.

Clinical signs

- Septicaemia and high temperature in piglets.
- Nervous signs
- Frail piglets at birth.
- Pneumonia.
- Head on one side.

Treatment

- Listeria is generally sensitive to penicillin and ampicillin.
- In outbreaks it is essential to recognize the sources of infection and lessen the exposure to them.

Tetanus

It is caused by Clostridium tetani, a bacteria that releases toxins that harm the central nervous system. The creature, which can create spores, resides in the large intestine. It can be found in the faeces of numerous mammals as well as in various soils. This disease can be an issue for pigs who live outside. The incubation time ranges from 1 to 10 weeks, with shorter intervals resulting in more severe illness. The sickness is infrequent in nursing piglets less than 2 weeks old.

Symptoms

- Hypersensitivity.
- Stiffness muscles.
- Stiff tail.
- Muscle spasms in ears and face.
- High mortality.
- Backward arching of head and neck

Prevention

- Once clinical indications appear, there is no effective treatment.
- Sow vaccination is really effective.
- Antitoxins are used during castration.
- When pigs with wounds exposed to soil, preventive antibiotics, particularly penicillin, are used.

Tuberculosis

Swine tuberculosis is now uncommon; however the Mycobacterium avium complex is the most frequent. In addition, the complex produces non-progressive, subclinical disorders in healthy individual. The biggest danger is that it could induce serious sickness in persons who are immunocompromised. In most nations, if lesions in the neck are identified in the slaughterhouse, the head is confiscated; if lesions are found in the mesenteric lymph nodes that flow into the intestines, the viscera are confiscated. If the sickness spreads throughout the body, which is uncommon, the entire carcass will be confiscated. Normal cooking of pork in the kitchen removes the organism if the minor lesions are not identified during inspection.

Symptoms

Small lumps form in the lymph nodes of the neck and those draining into the small intestine.

The vast majority of the time, the lesions are not progressive, do not spread throughout the body, and do not make the pig sick. They are not eliminated.

There are no clinical indications of infection, and there is no difference in productivity between infected and uninfected pigs.

Diagnosis

The tuberculin skin test is used to diagnose the disease in live pigs, although the producer usually discovers the disease is present on his farm when he receives the list of the proportion of seizures in the slaughterhouse.

Prevention

- There is no treatment in common.
- Remove contaminated feed and bedding.
- Use chlorinated water.

Ringworm

Ringworm (fungal infection) occurs in swine on occasion and can affect any age group. Although instances are mostly rare, occasional outbreaks affect a wide range of animals, particularly sows. The fungi Microsporum nanum or Trichophyton verrucosum cause the majority of ringworm. Ringworm is caused by several different species of fungi (called dermatophytes) infecting the skin of the pig. Ringworm is infrequent, albeit it is slightly more prevalent in outdoor pigs than in indoor pigs. It has little effect on pigs that appear to be ignorant of it. It goes away on its own after a month or two and is inconsequential.

Lesions can appear everywhere, but on older swine, they are most commonly observed on the neck or behind the ears. Ringworm lesions begin as brown spreading regions a few centimetres in diameter but can grow to be five to ten centimetres in diameter. Mature lesions have a core, brown crust, minimum or no hair loss, and are non-pruritic. Ringworm must be distinguished from sarcoptic mange in adult pigs, especially if lesions are located behind the ears. Ringworm must be distinguished from pityriasis rosea and exudative epidermitis ("greasy pig") in early growing pigs. Ringworm is usually diagnosed through microscopic analysis of skin scrapings or histopathologic investigation of skin lesions.

Ringworm is normally self-limiting; however lesions might take months to heal. During the winter, lesions are more common. Ringworm can be treated orally with nystatin or griseofulvin, although it is usually left alone to heal. People should be aware that ringworm is contagious.

Fungi

Fungi (moulds and yeasts) thrive in moist environments, such as poorly stored grains. Some species produce poisons (mycotoxins) during the proliferation process, which can cause a variety of clinical symptoms when consumed.

To prevent fungus from proliferating and creating poisons on the farm, the following things are critical.

- Never store soggy maize or grain.
- Avoid allowing grain to ferment.
- Inspect feed hoppers on a daily basis.
- Grain bins should be treated on a regular basis.
- Check holding bins for leaks on a monthly basis.
- Don't let feed go to waste or fester in feed troughs.
- Always double-check your basic feed ingredients.
- Before feeding, visually inspect the completed feed.

Fungi can also induce miscarriage or mastitis in individual pigs, but this is uncommon and has little overall significance.

Glossary

Abortion - The production of an early non-viable litter.

Agalactia - Failure of milk let down.

Belly – The underside of a pig.

Baconer – A pig reared to produce bacon. This is usually around 80-100kg, and reached between eight and ten months of age.

Bagging up – the enlarged size of the teats in preparation of milk production

Barrow – a male pig that is castrated before reaching sexual maturity.

Boar – a male pig over 6 months of age that can be used for breeding.

Breed – to permit a male and female animal to mate; a group of animals with the same characteristics and ancestry.

Castrate – to sterilize a male pig by removing the testicles.

Cervix - The neck of the womb.

Concentrates – a balanced dry feed in the form of pellets

Conception rate - As a % this is calculated by:

$$\frac{\text{No. of females which conceived x 100}}{\text{No. of females mated or inseminated}}$$

The calculation is based on a given period of time.

Conceptus - Fertilised ovum and embryo.

Corpora haemorrhagica - When the follicle ruptures to release the egg there is a little amount of haemorrhage. This is the name given to the bloody tissues that remain.

Corpus albucans - After pregnancy or after the animal has been in oestrus the corpus luteum disappears and shrinks to a tiny white body called the corpus albucans.

Corpus luteum - This is the body that produces progesterone, the female hormone that maintains pregnancy.

Cryptorchid - A male pig whose testes have not descended through the inguinal canals.

Cuts – the end products of pork after the butchering process is complete.

Cutter – A pig reared to produce larger joints of meat, ranging somewhere between 76 – 85 kg.

Dam – the female parent.

Dead weight – the given total weight of a pig after slaughter

Dewclaw – the small appendage just above the hoof on the posterior side.

Dressed weight – the weight of a pig carcass after it has been gutted and prepped for butchering.

Drift – a group of young pigs.

Drove – a herd or group of pigs.

Embryo - The multicellular organism that develops in the uterus from the fertilised egg up to about 20-30 days when it becomes a foetus.

Endometritis - Inflammation of the lining of the womb the endometrium.

Epididymis - A coiled tube attached to the upper surface of the testicle where the sperm is stored.

Erythema - Reddening of the skin that is often seen when one or more mammary glands have mastitis.

Estrus – when a female animal is in heat and ready to mate.

Farrow – to give birth

Farrowing rate (%) This equals

$$\frac{\text{No. females farrowed}}{\text{No. females mated}} \times 100$$

Fertilised ovum - The egg as it multiplies and grows to approximately day seven post fertilisation.

Finishing – the phase between when a pig is born and when it is ready to go to market.

Foetus - This explains the developing piglet from approximately 30 days through to maturity.

Forage – when pigs attain their own food by searching their environment.

Gestation – The length of a pregnancy.

Gilt – a young female pig that has never given birth.

Grower – a pig that is intended to be sold for slaughter.

Heterosis – the process of cross-breeding pigs to produce more favorable breed traits such as litter size, conception rate, piglet survival rate and growth.

Hock – the back leg joint.

Implantation - The attachment of the embryo to the uterine wall by establishment of the placenta commencing 12 to 14 days post-mating.

Inguinal canal - Gap between the muscles of the abdomen in the groin through which the spermatic cord passes from the abdomen to the testicle.

Irregular return - A return to oestrus more than 23 days after the previous one.

Jowl – the underside of a pig's neck.

Lactation length - The period from farrowing to weaning in days.

Leg – the leg of a pig from which ham is derived.

Litter – a group of piglets born to a single sow.

Loin – the muscles on either side of the spine which produces pork tenderloins.

Mammary oedema - Mammary tissues may contain excess amounts of fluid at farrowing.

Mastitis metritis agalactia syndrome (MMA) - This syndrome is most typically related with mastitis, namely coliform mastitis caused by E. coli or Klebsiella, but it is also linked to endometritis.

Mastitis - Inflammation of the mammary gland is invariably associated with infection.

Mating - The complete act of copulation involving one or more services.

Mummified pigs - Piglets which died in the uterus and in which the tissues and fluids have been reabsorbed leaving black shrunken skeletal remains.

Non productive days - These are any days when the sows and gilts are not pregnant or suckling.

Oestrus (or heat) - The period during which the sow is receptive to the boar. Usually 1-3 days.

Oestrus cycle - The period from one oestrus to another. 19-22 days interval is normal.

Orchitis - Inflammation of the testicle.

Ovaries - Two small structures which control the oestrus cycle and from which the follicles are produced and the eggs released.

Oxytocin - A hormone produced by the anterior pituitary gland. Its function is to release milk from the glands and at the same time cause the uterus to contract.

Parity - Used to describe the number of times a female has farrowed.

Pastern – the bone that connects the hoof and leg joints.

Pig creep – Highly palatable, easily digestible feed offered to piglets while suckling normally around 10 to 14 days of age

Piglet – young pig still suckling from the sow

Porker – A pig reared to produce pork. This is usually around 60kg, and reached between four and six months of age.

Processing – preparing a slaughtered animal for packaging or storage.

Prolactin - A hormone from the pituitary gland involved in the beginning and maintenance of milk production.

Pyometra - Accumulation of pus in the womb following infection.

Rear Flank – located between the ribs and stifle.

Regular return - A return to oestrus usually 19-22 days after previous one.

Returned service – Sow re-served after a previous unsuccessful mating.

Rooting – when pigs dig up the earth with their noses in search of food.

Rump – the area on a pig's back just above it's tail.

Runt – Smallet piglet in the litter

Salpingitis - Inflammation of the oviducts that carry the eggs from the ovary down towards the womb.

Scrotum - This is a sack made of relatively thin pliable skin which has a muscular inner fibro-elastic layer which contracts in a cold environment and relaxes in a hot environment.

Seminal vesicles - These are glands which together with the prostate and bulbo-urethral glands provide fluid and nourishment for the sperm, the fluids being passed out during ejaculation.

Service date – date of first mating during any one oestrus period.

Service – Mating within oestrus period.

Sire – the male parent.

Snout – a pig's nose.

Sow – an adult female pig that has farrowed a litter of piglets.

Spermatic cord - Fibrous cord, containing the vas deferens and blood vessels, by which the testicles are suspended.

Stag – a male pig that was castrated after reaching sexual maturity.

Stifle – the "knee" joint in the hind leg.

Stillborn pigs - Piglets observed dead at birth.

Testicle - The organ in which the sperm is produced.

Urethritis - inflammation of the urethra, the tube which carries both sperm and urine down the penis in the boar or urine from the bladder to the vagina in the sow.

Uterus - Consists of two horns upto 1.5m in length that contains the foetuses.

Vagina - The passageway from the exterior to the cervix.

Vaginitis - inflammation occurs following trauma, infection or multiple matings.

Vas deferens - The muscular tube that at ejaculation propels the sperm from the tail of the epididymis on the testes up through the inguinal canal and into the urethra where it joins just below the neck of the bladder.

Vasectomising - a boar involves cutting the vas deferens midway between the tail of the epididymis and its entry to the abdomen, removing 30-50mm of it.

Vulva - The vagina opens to the exterior through the fleshy lips of the vulva.

Wallow – a muddy puddle pigs use to cool their body temperature in hot weather.

Wean – to transition an animal from its mother's milk to adult food.

Weaner – piglets separated from the sow at eight weeks and no longer feeding from the sow